Morphodynamic imaging in Achalasia

This book embarks on a journey never taken before, approaching the imaging of the disease of achalasia with new pathophysiological assumptions in mind, coming from the Chicago Classification of Manometric Diagnosis. Using state-of-the-art, modern X-ray technology, the authors have developed a schematic and simple approach to detection, diagnosis, and patient stadiation and prognostic stratification for radiologists, clinicians, and students.

Key Features:

1. Serves as a useful guide to structured and comprehensive reporting of barium swallows, both in achalasia and other esophageal motility disorders.
2. Allows radiologists, specialists, and trainees to comprehensively understand achalasia from anatomic, pathophysiologic, therapeutic points of view, allowing for exact comprehension, detection, and reporting of the radiologic hallmarks of the disease.
3. Empowers readers to diagnose and define the exact achalasia subtype in each patient, due to the specifically developed Fatebenefratelli (FBF) score.

Morphodynamic Imaging in Achalasia

Edited by Giovanni Fontanella

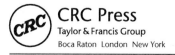

CRC Press
Taylor & Francis Group
Boca Raton London New York

CRC Press is an imprint of the
Taylor & Francis Group, an **informa** business

First edition published 2023
by CRC Press
6000 Broken Sound Parkway NW, Suite 300, Boca Raton, FL 33487-2742

and by CRC Press
4 Park Square, Milton Park, Abingdon, Oxon, OX14 4RN

CRC Press is an imprint of Taylor & Francis Group, LLC

Library of Congress Cataloging-in-Publication Data
Names: Fontanella, Giovanni, editor.
Title: Morphodynamic imaging in achalasia / edited by Giovanni Fontanella.
Description: First edition. | Boca Raton : CRC Press, 2023. | Includes bibliographical references and index.
Identifiers: LCCN 2022028592 (print) | LCCN 2022028593 (ebook) | ISBN 9781032335858 (hardback) |
    ISBN 9781032335841 (paperback) | ISBN 9781003320302 (ebook)
Subjects: MESH: Esophageal Achalasia—diagnostic imaging | Fluoroscopy | Barium Sulfate
Classification: LCC RC815.7 (print) | LCC RC815.7 (ebook) | NLM WI 258 | DDC 616.3/207572—
    dc23/eng/20221026
LC record available at https://lccn.loc.gov/2022028592
LC ebook record available at https://lccn.loc.gov/2022028593

ISBN: 978-1-032-33585-8 (hbk)
ISBN: 978-1-032-33584-1 (pbk)
ISBN: 978-1-003-32030-2 (ebk)

DOI: 10.1201/9781003320302

Typeset in Times
by Apex CoVantage, LLC

Contents

Preface

One of the directions I reckon that the scientific progress and research should always follow is that of the unknown. No progress can actually be defined as such without an initial step, sometimes even a tiny one, into the unknown. Of course, when selecting the matter of research, many factors have to be taken into account, some of them being quite limiting. In my case, I cannot recall the exact moment I started researching on achalasia—it just started, somehow, in a moment in the past, after my first encounter with this disease, some 15 years ago. I have always had a soft spot for little known or rare diseases, those that you are most likely not to encounter in a whole career. Achalasia was presented to me as a rare disease, and it still is, but I have always been exposed to clinical environments in which patients with this condition were more frequent than normal. This means I had the chance to talk to them, take their clinical history, feel the actual discomfort or pain they felt, and understand the psychological issues that achalasia inflicted on them. This experience most likely was etched somehow on my mind and stimulated me to walk in the direction of the unknown, or perhaps, little known of achalasia. The rare disease became real people, not more nor less important than those affected by other conditions, but very worthy of research and clinical attention. This simple collection of frames and notes, written primarily for myself, kept growing during the years, until it reached the final form you are now holding in your hands.

I sincerely hope you do appreciate our efforts towards a better clinical knowledge of this condition.

Giovanni Fontanella, MD FRSA

Acknowledgements

I would like, first and foremost, to express my gratitude to the Most Compassionate and Most Merciful, the One that enabled myself to be in the world, through the grace of the best parents one can possibly desire, Mirella and Eugenio. I would not be in the position I am now, had it not been for their patience and constant, daily guidance towards hard work and humility. The foundations of everything I do lie in both of them.

I am immensely thankful to the person who has been my everything for the last few years, Simona—without her, I would not be here right now. She helps me to be a better person, to strive towards a better future and do what I love, and she does so by example. Her influence and support in the making of this book have been tremendous: editing and writing of the technical section are hers, and so are some of the anatomical and technical drawings.

Thank you to my furry daughter, Ivana, teacher of unconditional love.

It would be impossible to cite here all the important figures I have met in my professional life and who, knowingly or not, somehow changed my life, my beliefs, my way of thinking and working. One of them is prof. Gina Brown, whose research has been inspirational in my formation years and still is to this very day—to her goes our sincere gratitude for writing a foreword for this monograph.

Sincere thanks go to Biondo Francesco Giuseppe, Giuseppe Fuggi, Francesca Russo, Rocco Granata and all the contributors for their expertise and invaluable help in making this volume.

A huge thank you goes to Giovanni Limone, one of the few remaining craftsmen of barium imaging—the images he produces are not only of invaluable diagnostic quality but also unique pieces of didactic art.

Last but not least, thank you to my hospital, Sacro Cuore di Gesù, in Benevento, Italy, and to the wider family of the Brothers Hospitaliers of Saint John of God/Fatebenefratelli, to whom the FBF score is dedicated.

Giovanni Fontanella, MD FRSA

Foreword

It is a tremendous honour for me to be invited to write the foreword to this excellent monograph. In my opinion, adding to the body of knowledge through the detailed study of disease and a desire to improve the lives of patients through well-conducted research is a fundamental part of what makes us good doctors.

This thesis illustrates what can be archived by a disciplined and structured analysis of commonplace imaging. The technique of fluoroscopy has been in existence since the 1950s—yet this volume illustrates how much was not known and still is to be understood by careful attention to detail of barium swallow images and videofluoroscopic techniques.

There is much to learn from reading this book. First, an appreciation that physiology is crucial and almost uniquely visualized in vivo by videofluoroscopic technique. Second, that experience and study of Achalasia provides new insights and a greater understanding of both the physiologic and pathologic impact of this disease.

The detailed anatomic, physiologic and histopathologic documentation of observed disease processes has been behind most of the major advances we see in medicine. Furthermore, enabling others to learn and understand new observations and concepts and providing a structure to improve imaging interpretation as described in this work are also critical.

Videofluoroscopy and barium imaging have been in existence for many decades, but "The real voyage of discovery consists not in seeking new landscapes but in having new eyes" (Marcel Proust, 1923). I congratulate Dr Fontanella in taking this journey of discovery in this rare but important disease.

Prof. Gina Brown, MBBS MD MRCP FRCR FASCRS (Hon)
Professor of GI Radiology and Consultant Radiologist
Imperial College London

Editor Biography

Giovanni Fontanella, MD FRSA, is an abdominal and gastrointestinal consultant radiologist based in Benevento, Italy, at the Sacro Cuore di Gesù—Fatebenefratelli Hospital. His alma mater is the historical Vanvitelli University in Naples, Italy, one of the most important schools for gastrointestinal imaging in Italy. The interest for GI and abdominal imaging was consolidated at the prestigious St. Mark's Hospital in London, United Kingdom, a competitive and top-level environment. In Benevento, he conducts both clinical activity and research, with the focus on constant testing, innovation, and optimization of all imaging techniques to the needs of the clinical practice. He is currently working on further developments of gel-enhanced MR fistulography, which was entirely developed and used in clinical routine for the first time at the Fatebenefratelli Hospital; morphodynamic imaging techniques in pharyngoesophageal motility diseases; and virtual colonoscopy. His academic record stands, at the time of writing, at 26 top-level publications, most of them in the field of GI imaging, with several participations as a speaker at international radiology meetings, such as the European Congress of Radiology (ECR 2019, 2020, 2021), Congress of the European Society of Gastrointestinal and Abdominal Imaging (ESGAR 2019, 2020), and Annual Radiology Meeting in Dubai (2020, 2021). Dr Fontanella is a member of several radiology societies worldwide, such as the European Society of Radiology, European Society of Gastrointestinal and Abdominal Imaging, British Society of Gastrointestinal and Abdominal Imaging, Radiological Society of North America, and Korean Society of Radiology. He regularly hosts GI-themed seminars for the Radiological Society of the Emirates. In 2021, Dr Fontanella was nominated Fellow of the Royal Society of Arts in London.

Contributors

Carmine Augusto Tommaso Manganiello
Ospedale Sacro Cuore di Gesù, FBF
Benevento, Italy

Simona Borrelli
UPMC Hillman Cancer Center
'Villa Maria'
Mirabella Eclano, Italy

Barbara Brogna
A.O.R.N. S.G. Moscati
Avellino, Italy

Sandro Calderazzo
Ospedale Sacro Cuore di Gesù, FBF
Benevento, Italy

Simone Coviello
Ospedale Sacro Cuore di Gesù, FBF
Benevento, Italy

Silvio De Lucia
Ospedale Sacro Cuore di Gesù, FBF
Benevento, Italy

Felice De Rosa
Ospedale Sacro Cuore di Gesù, FBF
Benevento, Italy

Diego De Stasio
Ospedale Sacro Cuore di Gesù, FBF
Benevento, Italy

Anna Vincenza De Lucia
Ospedale Sacro Cuore di Gesù, FBF
Benevento, Italy

Parente Emilio
Ospedale Sacro Cuore di Gesù, FBF
Benevento, Italy

Pacifico Fabio
Ospedale Sacro Cuore di Gesù, FBF
Benevento, Italy

Giuliano Fabrizio
Ospedale Sacro Cuore di Gesù, FBF
Benevento, Italy

Andrea Festa
Ospedale Sacro Cuore di Gesù, FBF
Benevento, Italy

Giuseppe Fuggi
Ospedale Sacro Cuore di Gesù, FBF
Benevento, Italy

Micco Gianfranco
Ospedale Sacro Cuore di Gesù, FBF
Benevento, Italy

Ferdinando Giorgione
Ospedale Sacro Cuore di Gesù, FBF
Benevento, Italy

Fuggi Giovanni
Ospedale Sacro Cuore di Gesù, FBF
Benevento, Italy

Biondo Francesco Giuseppe
Ospedale Sacro Cuore di Gesù, FBF
Benevento, Italy

Rocco Granata
A.O. 'San Pio'
Benevento, Italy

Antonietta Iarriccio
Ospedale Sacro Cuore di Gesù, FBF
Benevento, Italy

Russo Maurizio
Ospedale Sacro Cuore di Gesù, FBF
Benevento, Italy

Saverio Mazzeo
Ospedale Sacro Cuore di Gesù, FBF
Benevento, Italy

Carlo Nazzaro
Ospedale Sacro Cuore di Gesù, FBF
Benevento, Italy

Maurizio Orso
Ospedale Sacro Cuore di Gesù, FBF
Benevento, Italy

Francesca Russo
A.O. 'San Pio'
Benevento, Italy

Marco Russo
Ospedale Sacro Cuore di Gesù, FBF
Benevento, Italy

Dello Iacono Umberto
Ospedale Buon Consiglio, FBF
Naples, Italy

Abbreviations

AP	anteroposterior
CECT	contrast enhanced computed tomography
CNS	central nervous system
CT	computed tomography
DCI	distal contractile integral
EGD	esophagogastroduodenoscopy
EGJ	esophagogastric junction
GABA	*gamma*-aminobutyric acid
GERD	gastroesophageal reflux disease
GI	gastrointestinal
Gy	gray
HLA	human leukocyte antigen
HPV	human papilloma virus
HRM	high-resolution manometry
HSV	herpes simplex virus
IFN	interferon
IL	interleukin
IRP	integrated relaxation pressure
JCV	John Cunningham virus
kV	kilovolts
LES	lower esophageal sphincter
LHM	laparoscopic Heller myotomy
LPO	left posterior oblique
mA	milliampere
MDT	multidisciplinary team
MEN	multiple endocrine neoplasia
NKs	natural killer cells
NO	nitric oxide
PACS	picture archiving and communication system
PD	pneumatic dilation
PED	primary esophageal dilation
POEM	peroral endoscopic myotomy
RAO	right anterior oblique
RIS	radiological information system
RL	right lateral
RPO	right posterior oblique
SLE	systemic lupus erythematosus
SNP	single nucleotide polymorphism
TIMPs	matrix proteinases and inhibitors

TTR	transthyretin
UES	upper esophageal sphincter
VIP	vasoactive intestinal peptide
VZV	varicella zoster virus

Introduction

After 40 years spent as a surgeon dedicated to the treatment of surgical diseases of the esophagus, I am very pleased to write this introduction to a work that comes out of the passion and radiological expertise of my colleague, Dr Giovanni Fontanella, who has shown that he has made great use of the experience acquired, even in a niche sector of medicine.

During the last 20 years, with the help of new technologies, knowledge of great importance has been achieved on pathophysiology, etiopathogenesis, diagnosis and therapy, in the field of functional diseases of the esophagus, and, in particular, in acalasia. These interesting developments have encouraged and induced the author to write this excellent monograph with an interdisciplinary spirit, such as to make the reading of the text interesting for all specialists and connoisseurs of the subject, because it is aimed to complete their knowledge. The scarcity of experience, due to the rarity of achalasia, whose incidence per year stands at 0.5–1.2 per 100,000 inhabitants, makes it even more necessary today to publish a complete monograph that can be referred to. It is enriched with both new and important data from the literature, and recent common clinical experiences had at the Sacro Cuore di Gesù Hospital, Fatebenefratelli, in Benevento, Italy.

Dr Fontanella's specific merit in this book is of having focused, developed and expanded, in the radiological field, the concept of "morphodynamical imaging". This contributes in a simpler and clearer way to the diagnostic clarification of esophageal disease already in the first phase of the radiological study, also allowing us surgeons an immediate understanding of the evolutionary stage of achalasic disease and its therapeutic orientation. The author has also developed the "FBF Achalasia Scoring System", which consists of an original and systematic classification of the disease, not only based on the morphology of the esophagus, as done in classic radiology texts, but also on the dynamic findings observed during the radiological study with barium, taking into account only five parameters. The FBF Achalasia Scoring System, since its conception, has proved to be in complete agreement with the Chicago Classification and the more modern H R i M classification. In clinical practice, this allows the Upper GI MDT to speak a common language and to integrate diagnosis and therapy earlier, in a simpler way.

However, it is impossible to end this introduction without thanking our common patients, both those we remember and those we have forgotten, for having entrusted their lives to us, offering us the opportunity to acquire part of the experience reported in the book.

Biondo Francesco Giuseppe, MD

Historic Overview of Achalasia

Giovanni Fontanella and Simona Borrelli

Contents

1.1 INTRODUCTION

Sir Thomas Willis, the preeminent anatomist of the time, perhaps better known for the description of the eponymous endocranic vascular circle, published one of the earliest descriptions of achalasia in 1674 (Figure 1.1). Willis was not only the first to describe a case of probable achalasia, but he was also the first to devise a reasonable treatment modality that allowed patients to support themselves for a period of at least 15 years, namely using a "whalebone staff with a button of sponge". Following his original description of the condition, achalasia has been known by a variety of terms, including cardiospasm, megaesophagus, diffuse dilation of the esophagus without stenosis, and idiopathic dilation of the esophagus. Sir Arthur Hurst coined the term achalasia, which is derived from the Greek word ἀχάλασις, which means "lack of relaxation" or "inability to relax". Achalasia is, in fact, a condition that affects the ability to relax of the lower esophageal sphincter. However, it is unclear when Hurst came up with the term "achalasia", but he did so in a monograph published as early as 1915. Hurst gives credit for the invention of the term to Sir Cooper Perry, then superintendent at the Guy's Hospital in London, who was at the time the author of this monograph. Initially, Hurst objected to the term "cardiospasm" because it implied an active, abnormal spasm of the cardia, which he believed was in opposition to his theory of the disease's pathogenesis, which was one of normal muscular contraction hampered by a loss of neuromuscular inhibition near the esophagogastric junction. Despite the fact that achalasia is now the widely accepted term to describe the

DOI: 10.1201/9781003320302-1

clinical entity, authors as early as 1964 proposed terms such as aganglionic achalasia and amyenteric achalasia in an attempt to incorporate the concepts of impaired esophageal peristalsis as well as impaired relaxation of the sphincter into the name. Theories about the origins of achalasia have been as diverse as the terms used to describe the condition itself. Hoffman described the condition as a psychogenic illness caused by "irrational love" and "uncontrollable desires" in 1733, and it has been around ever since. Other authors, such as Thieding, Weiss, and Winkelstein, have proposed that psychiatric therapy plays a significant role in the treatment of patients suffering from achalasia. The pathologic basis of

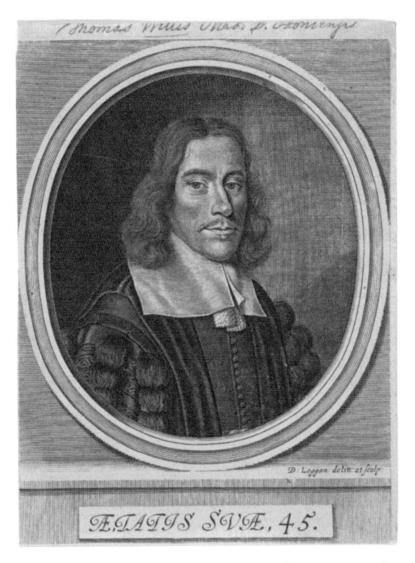

FIGURE 1.1   Portrait of Sir Thomas Willis, by David Logan, Rijksmuseum Amsterdam.

Source: Public domain image.

the disease, according to early investigators such as Purton and Hannay, was believed to be primary esophageal dilation (PED). Following the development of these theories, the theory of a hypertonic cardiac sphincter gradually took over. Von Mikulicz coined the term cardiospasm in the nineteenth century, and the term became widely accepted as more cases were reported in the rapidly expanding medical literature during the following century (Figure 1.2). When he published his findings in 1904, he estimated that over 100 cases had been reported. He was also the first to draw attention to the actual anatomic junction between the esophagus and stomach as the most likely site of physiologic dysfunction. The most succinct and comprehensive explanation of this theory was provided by Sturtevant in 1933, who defined cardiospasm as follows: "a condition in which, in the absence of any demonstrable obstructive pathologic change and usually without pain, food does not pass readily from the esophagus into the stomach but is retained in the esophagus, which, in the majority of cases, undergoes dilation, sometimes extreme".

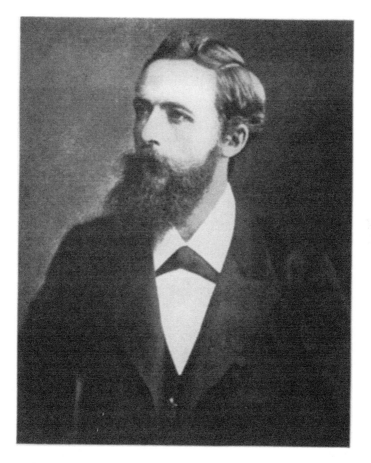

FIGURE 1.2   Johannes von Mikulicz.

Source: Public domain image.

Although spasm of the cardia was the most widely accepted theory of achalasia for a long time, it was not universally accepted, and other investigators came up with a variety of alternative explanations for the apparent gastroesophageal obstruction. One prominent school of thought held that the apparent esophageal stenosis was the result of a physical obstruction in the esophagus. Mosher described the classic clinical and radiographic findings of achalasia in 1922 and asserted that the condition was caused by a "tunnel" of liver through which the esophagus travels prior to its anastomosis with the stomach, which he believed to be the case. Breathing and swallowing were said to be disordered in affected patients, resulting in the food bolus in the esophagus meeting a closed region created by the movement of the liver and its effects on the diaphragmatic hiatus, according to the doctor. A physical obstruction, according to Chevalier Jackson, the father of otorhinolaryngology, was also suspected of being responsible. An esophageal obstruction, according to Jackson, is caused by a diaphragmatic "pinchcock". He asserted that it was a normal mechanism responsible for the prevention of free regurgitation of stomach contents and that it was defined by the kinking of the distal esophagus caused by the action of the diaphragmatic crura in response to a full stomach. According to Jackson, the inability of the "pinchcock" to open was the cause of the dysphagia and esophageal dilation that were observed in patients with the condition. The condition was referred to as phrenoesophagospasm by the doctor who diagnosed it. In addition to the esophageal fibrosis theory, other theories of mechanical obstruction, such as the narrowing of the diaphragmatic hiatus, were popular and remain popular today. On the other hand, Hurst's argument that tonic spasm of the cardia was unlikely to be the true cause of achalasia because of the lack of cardiac muscular hypertrophy on dissection gave rise to the contemporary theory about the cause of achalasia. He hypothesized that achalasia was the clinical manifestation of a loss of normal inhibition of the distal esophagus and that it should be classified as neuromuscular dysfunction rather than muscular spasm to be more appropriately classified. During his research in 1927, he discovered a pronounced fibrocellular infiltrate and loss of normal neuronal structure in distal esophageal ganglion cells of Auerbach's plexus, which is located in the region of the lower esophageal sphincter (abdominal wall). Hurst and Rake were among the first to demonstrate a correlation between the pathology and histology of the condition. Even though Hurst was responsible for naming achalasia and receiving most of the credit for unraveling the disease's pathogenesis, he was not the first to propose that the failure of the lower esophageal sphincter to relax was the primary abnormality involved. In 1888, at two separate meetings, Einhorn and Meltzer proposed that one possible explanation for the symptom complex seen in achalasia was a failure of the normal relaxation at the distal esophagus or cardia, respectively. When Rolleston proposed that impaired esophageal relaxation was responsible for the progressively worsening dysphagia and dilation seen in the condition in 1896, he was considered a revolutionary thinker. However, it was not until the late twentieth century that impaired lower esophageal sphincter inhibition was widely accepted as a cause of the condition. In 1949, various investigators, including Kramer and Ingelfinger, were employing esophageal balloon kymograph motility methods to investigate cardiospasm. They claimed that the distal esophageal spasm was only one aspect of a larger, more generalized esophageal motor disorder; however, it is unclear whether they were actually examining patients with achalasia during their studies. It was not until the 1960s and 1970s, when detailed anatomic analysis combined with advanced histopathologic techniques demonstrated the loss of inhibitory neurons in the lower esophageal sphincter, that the tonic contraction of the lower esophageal sphincter became widely recognized as the primary cause of the condition. Achalasia continues to be a disease that is poorly understood, both in terms of its etiology and in terms of the most effective treatment strategies. Since Willis's first description of achalasia 400 years ago, there has been an exponential increase in our understanding of the species. Unfortunately, it appears that each new answer to a question about the disease is followed by a new round of questions. The development of endoscopic technology, which was largely influenced by the otorhinolaryngology community in the early twentieth century, has been the most significant technological advance that has allowed us to gain a better understanding of the condition. Endoscopy allowed for direct observation of the esophagus, as well as the taking of biopsies and the placement of dilators through a natural route. As a result of the advancement of esophageal manometry and the improvement of histopathology techniques, the functional and anatomic evidence of esophageal abnormalities associated with achalasia have been provided in greater numbers and with greater clarity.

1.2 FURTHER READING

Adams HD: Amyenteric achalasia of the esophagus. *Surg Gynecol Obstet* 119:251, 1964

Barrett NR, Franklin RH: Concerning the unfavourable late results of certain operations performed in the treatment of cardiospasm. *Br J Surg* 37:194, 1949

Einhorn M: A case of dysphagia with dilatation of the oesophagus. *Med Rec* 34:751, 1888

Ellis FH, Olsen AM: *Achalasia of the Esophagus.* Philadelphia, WB Saunders, 1969

Freeman L: An operation for the relief of cardiospasm associated with dilatation and tortuosity of the esophagus. *Ann Surg* 78:173, 1923

Gottstein G: Technik und klinik der oesopagoskopie. *Mitt Grenzgeb Med Chir* 8:57, 1901

Gottstein G: Weitere Forttschritte in der Therapie des chronischen Cardiospasmus (mitsackartiger Erweiterung der Speiserohre). *Verh Dtsch Ges Chir* 37:470, 1908

Hannay AJ: An extraordinary dilatation (with hypertrophy?) of all the thoracic portion of the oesophagus causing dysphagia. *Endinb Med Surg J* 40:65, 1833

Hurst AF: Achalasia of the cardia. *Q J Med* 8:300, 1915

Hurst AF: The treatment of achalasia of the cardia. *Lancet* 1:618, 1927

Hurst AF, Rake GW: Achalasia of the cardia (so-called cardiospasm). *Q J Med* 23:491, 1930

Jackson C: The diaphragmatic pinchcock in so-called cardiospasm. *Laryngoscope* 32:139, 1922

Kramer P, Ingelfinger FJ: Cardiospasm, a generalized disorder of esophageal motility. *Am J Med* 7:174, 1949

Kummel H: Zur Operation des Kardiospasmus und des Oesophaguscarcinoms. *Arch Kiln Chir* 117:193, 1921

Lotheissen G. Cited by Von Hacker V, Lotheissen G: Chirurgie der Speiserohre. In Von Bruns P (ed): *Neue Deutsche Chirurgie*, vol 34. Stuttgart, Ferdinand Enke, 1926, p 281

Meltzer SG: Ein Fall von Dysphagie nebst Bemeerkungen. *Berlin Klin Wschr* 25:140, 1888

Meyer W: Impermeable cardiospasm successfully treated by thoracotomy and esophagoplication. *JAMA* 56:1437, 1911

Mosher HP: Liver tunnel and cardiospasm. *Laryngoscope* 32:348, 1922

Plummer HS: Diffuse dilatation of the esophagus without anatomic stenosis. *JAMA* 58:2013, 1912

Pribram BO: Zur Pathologie und Chirurgie der spastischen Neurosen. *Arch Klin Chir* 120:207, 1922

Purton T: An extraordinary case of distension of the oesophagus, forming a sac, extending from two inches below the pharynx to the cardiac orifice of the stomach. *London Med Phys J* 46:540, 1821

Ripley HR, Olsen AM, Kirklin JW: Esophagitis after esophagogastric anastamosis. *Surgery* 32:1, 1952

Rolleston HD: Simple dilatation of the oesophagus. *Trans Path Soc (London)* 47:37, 1896

Russel JC: Diagnosis and treatment of spasmodic stricture of the esophagus. *BMJ* 1:1450, 1898

Sturtevant M: Cardiospasm: with a review of the literature. *Arch Intern Med* 51:714, 1933

Thieding F: Ueber cardiospasmus. Atonie und "idiopathische" dilatation der Speisorohre. *Bruns Beitr Kiln Chir* 121:237, 1921

Von Mikulicz J: Zur pathologie und therapie des cardiospasmus. *Munchen Med Wechnchr* 30:17, 1904

Evolution of Fluoroscopy and Barium Swallow

2

Simona Borrelli

Contents

2.1 INTRODUCTION

The barium swallow examination has evolved since its inception at the beginning of the twentieth century, from being considered a rather primitive evaluation of the swallowing function to what is today considered a comprehensive imaging modality that allows the specialist physician to assess both anatomy and function of the oral cavity, pharynx and oesophagus. Our way of describing this is simplified into the words 'morphodynamic imaging' that, appropriately, also make up the title of this book; this definition, used rather tentatively at first and especially during our radiology training, should not

DOI: 10.1201/9781003320302-2

be thought of just a pointless way of describing the act of acquiring moving images. A definition is needed to establish, in a clear way, the existence and the importance of an imaging modality that has, albeit in different forms, always been there and can now achieve great results and clinical relevance. The greatness of barium swallow is that it is a widely available, rather inexpensive, non-invasive test with which a wide host of pharyngoesophageal morphologic and functional abnormalities can be diagnosed. Technologic innovations often tend to shadow the importance and usefulness of what, still to this very day, is a basic examination that guides clinical or surgical decisions. Even though our objective with this book is to project barium swallow into the future, giving it a different dimension and making extensive use, ironically enough, of technologic innovations, in the next few pages, we will describe the constantly changing and evolving role of imaging in the diagnosis of pharyngoesophageal diseases in the last century, by recalling the evolution of fluoroscopic equipment, radiography and, last but not least, barium-based contrast media.

2.2 FROM FLUOROSCOPY TO MODERN IMAGING

While radiography is a technique that essentially acquires static images, by capturing a continuous set of X-ray images, fluoroscopy allows us to assess morphodynamical anatomy real-time, in vivo (Figure 2.1). Another difference between radiography and fluoroscopy is that the latter has less intrinsic contrast and space resolution but, at the same time, a much lower radiation dose per second. Considering a 22.83 cm field-of-view, radiation dose for fluoroscopy is 0.2–0.3 IGy, while the radiation dose for radiography is much higher at 5–10 IGy. However, a basic principle of fluoroscopy is continuous radiation, while only an instantaneous exposure is needed to produce a spot radiograph; in the end, in a barium swallow examination, the cumulative radiation dose of the fluoroscopy and that of the number of spot radiographs taken are substantially comparable, because it has been estimated that five to ten spot radiographs hold the same radiation dose of a minute of fluoroscopy at 30 frames per second. In the early twentieth century, barium swallows were carried out with primitive fluoroscopes, using a fluorescent screen and an X-ray tube, with the patient placed in-between. Usually, the fluoroscopist positioned himself or herself by facing the screen, protected by a leaded glass to decrease his or her own radiation exposure. The first fluorescent screens were coated with barium platinocyanide and later with cadmium tungstate or zinc cadmium sulfide. The contact between the X-rays passing through the patient and the coating resulted in the emission of very dim visible light, which forced the fluoroscopist to wear special glasses, dark- or red-adapted, to be able to adequately view the produced image. Of course, this rather primitive radiographic equipment was able to produce early radiographs, by making the X-rays passing through the patient react with a silver emulsion coating a plate of glass, hence the term 'flat plate' that is still colloquially and erroneously used today. A major innovation for both fluoroscopy and radiography was the development and subsequent introduction of image intensifiers, during the early 1950s. These devices allowed an electronic magnification of the output of

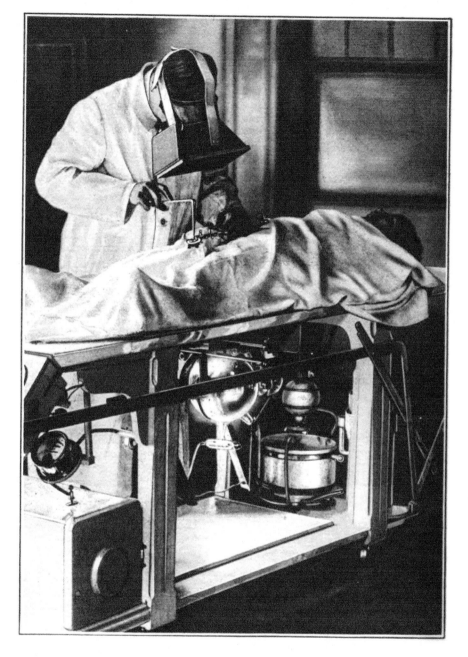

FIGURE 2.1   Surgical operation during World War I using a fluoroscope to find embedded bullets, 1917.

Source: M. Jungmann, "X-rays: Samaritans of war" in Waldemar Kaempffert, Ed., *The Book of Modern Marvels*, Leslie Judge Co., New York, p. 172—Public domain image.

fluorescent screens, dramatically improving the image-viewing experience. Conventional image intensifiers have been, even though much more recently, replaced by flat panel displays. We think it is of utmost importance to know where we come from and before going forwards, we will now briefly go through all these steps of the evolution from the inception of fluoroscopy to modern-day imaging.

2.3 IMAGE INTENSIFIER CHAIN

2.3.1 Generator

A generator is a device needed to produce an electric current, at a specified voltage (kVp) and current (mA), which is then sent to the X-ray tube. While 'continuous fluoroscopy' needs a continuous current, 'pulsed' fluoroscopy needs just short pulses of current (3–10 ms in length). Blurring artefacts due to motion can be minimized by using short exposure pulses.

2.3.2 X-ray Tube

Electric current produced from the generator is made to pass through a heated filament, in order to generate electrons, that are subsequently sent towards a positively charged tungsten anode. X-rays are created by making the electrons strike the so-called focal spot, a focal portion on the anode. The focal spot used for fluoroscopy, to improve geometric sharpness, is much smaller than that used for radiography; that is why radiography needs a much greater number of X-rays, a larger focal spot allowing greater tube currents to generate, minimizing tube heating (Figure 2.2)

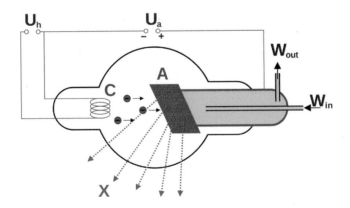

FIGURE 2.2   Coolidge side-window tube (scheme) C: filament/cathode (–) A: anode (+) W_{in} and W_{out}: water inlet and outlet of the cooling device.

2.3.3 Collimator

To reduce the amount of exposed tissue and, of course, decrease the radiation dose to the patient, radiopaque shutters are put in place to alter the shape of the X-ray beam. At the same time, this results in image contrast improvement.

2.3.4 Image Intensifier

An image intensifier is used to capture X-ray images converting them into visible light. Even though image intensifiers are progressively being replaced by new technology, namely flat panels fluoroscopes, they have been used since the early '50s and can still be found in many fluoroscopy practices and operating theatres. What happens in an image intensifier is that the X-rays passing through the patient reach a thin titanium called the input plate of the intensifier. The emission of light happens when the X-rays strike the inner surface of the plate and its fluorescent coating, which is generally made of cesium iodide; the light then proceeds to generate electrodes by hitting a photocathode layer of antimony. The electrons are subsequently accelerated from the photocathode toward the output phosphor, the electron beam being shaped by focusing electrodes and collimated onto an output phosphor plate. The visible image is the result of the energy conversion generated by the electrons striking the output plate (Figure 2.3).

2.3.5 Output Phosphor Image Displays

Early fluoroscopes were rather unpractical because to view the output image, a lens and mirror system was needed; moreover, light adaptation of the observer for viewing the

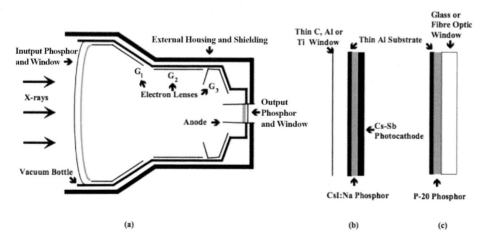

FIGURE 2.3   Schematic of an X-ray image intensifier.

Source: Public domain image.

green-yellow phosphor screen was needed, until, in the 1950s, closed-circuit television was developed and used as a superior method for displaying fluoroscopic images. The visible output phosphor image was converted by a television camera into an electronic signal, which was in turn sent directly to a cathode-ray television monitor for viewing. Of course, the result of using this analog television system was that the spatial resolution was reduced to about 1–2 line pairs per mm. The development of a charged couple device camera containing a solid state array of light sensors enabled the images to be stored as digital pixels that could be displayed on a liquid crystal digital monitor with a 1000–2500 matrix size. Returning to early fluoroscopes, another way of recording the images from the output phosphor was to use a roll of film by a Photospot camera. The film had then to be processed in a dark room, and the roll (or selected cut images from the roll) could finally be analyzed by the observer. A dynamical assessment was possible only by analyzing the rapid sequences of static images. In vivo, real-time fluoroscopy finally became possible when video recorder devices were developed, allowing the analysis of anatomic motion at normal speed or in slow motion, a great improvement for the interpretation of movement in comparison to what we have described before.

2.3.6 Radiographic Image Displays

Radiographic images used to be captured using analog fluoroscopic equipment, by manually loading film-screen cassettes into the fluoroscopic unit, exposing the film-screen combination, and then unloading the exposed cassette, only for a new cassette to be loaded and used for another exposure. When in need of rapid sequence images that, however, never could and never will replace a real-time continuous image, one could expose various portions of the cassette to the X-ray beam, obtaining two-on-one or three-on-one spot films. Of course, old fashion film-screen cassettes required darkrooms where the exposed films could be processed, back-lit viewers for spot-film analysis and file rooms for film storage. Cineradiography was the first technique used for real-time acquisition of radiographic images: rapid sequences of radiographs were recorded on 15- or 35-mm film in a movie camera, which had previously been installed in the fluoroscopic unit. The film was then obviously processed in a darkroom, then made to run through a movie projector, so that image analysis was actually performed on a movie screen. Even though this technique had better spatial and contrast resolution in comparison with fluoroscopic images, the whole processing and reviewing was inconvenient and, most importantly, associated with a higher radiation dose to the patient. The final blow that terminated cineradiography was the development of videotape machines, allowing fluoroscopy to be continuously recorded; video systems were, moreover, a lot easier to use. Another huge imaging revolution was the introduction, in the 1990s, of digital radiography that aimed to replace fluoroscopy and analog radiography, enabling much faster acquisition of radiographic and fluoroscopic images. Even though digital images had, of course, less spatial resolution (digital radiographs: 3.5–6 line pairs per mm; analog radiographs: 6–8 line pairs per mm), they had greater contrast resolution. Not needing physical storage like conventional films, digital images are transmitted electronically to a computer-based picture archiving communications system, the so-called PACS, from which they can be selectively retrieved to be viewed and interpreted on high-resolution monitors at computerized workstations. The adjustment of image brightness or contrast, with magnification of particular areas of interest, annotations of image findings for better interpretation and reporting of studies are possible through the post-processing. Digital imaging and the use of PACS systems eliminate the need for the production and storage of radiographic films, producing very profitable cost savings. The usage of digital fluoroscopic units is particularly convenient for a wide array of factors: first, shorter exposure times that translate in lower radiation exposure for the patient allowed by the instant display of images on fluoroscopy monitors; second, the shorter exposure also helps decrease motion artefacts and blurring, something of uttermost importance when considering pharyngoesophageal imaging. Also very convenient is that digital imaging does not require manual loading and unloading of cassettes, something that is normally done on analog fluoroscopic units, enabling a very fast image acquisition, considerably shortening the whole procedure duration. This is very important especially for the morphodynamical study of the pharyngoesophageal tract and, as we will see, for some forms of achalasia, too, especially considering that a swallowed bolus of barium traverses the pharynx and cervical esophagus approximately ten times faster than the thoracic esophagus. Image acquisition speed, however, is still not fast enough to display motion accurately, because modern digital imaging system enable to capture a maximum of eight images per second.

2.3.7 Flat Panel Fluoroscopes

When compared to an image intensifier, a flat panel fluoroscope is something quite different. X-rays passing through the patient are captured by a large array of photodiode cells, subsequently the flat panel process to digitize the X-ray image. Current flat panels measure about 25–40 cm and generally contain from 1.5 to 5 million detectors. After the X-rays pass through the patient, they are made to hit the Cesium iodide scintillator layer of each detector; this generates light, in proportion to the amount of X-ray flux that then hits the photodiode/transistor layer of the detector. The change in charge of each photodiode is then read by the electronic portion of the detector. While the electronic detector proceeds to read each photodiode, row by row, the fluoroscope generates a digitized image, so that it can be displayed on a high-resolution monitor. Even though very much depending on the field-of-view and the number of raster lines on the monitor, many television systems have a spatial revolution ranging between 0.5 and 1.5 line pairs per mm, a value much lower than the 5 line pairs per mm, the spatial resolution of the output phosphor of a standard fluoroscope. Spatial resolution in flat panel displays is actually determined by the detector size, with a current limit of about 2.5–3 line pairs per mm; in comparison, spatial resolution for analogic radiography is 6–8 line pairs per mm. Flat panel detectors enable the depiction of extremely dense and radiolucent structures, much better than image intensifiers; at the same time, the dynamic range of flat panel detectors is higher than that of image intensifiers. As previously said, the spatial resolution of flat panels depends very much on detector size and is, at least theoretically, independent of the field of view. So, using smaller field of views, through collimation, we are able to select information from the central portion of the flat panel and subsequently view it on the entire monitor. Using larger field of views,

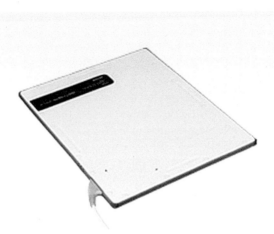

FIGURE 2.4 Flat panel fluoroscope.

Source: Public domain image.

data generation is so much higher that this forces the grouping of signals from four detectors. This reduces both data volume, spatial resolution and, at the same time, image mottle. Modern fluoroscopy can provide 30, 15, or 7.5 fluoroscopic frames per second and 2–4 radiographic images per second. Continuous motion is perceived by the eye at 30 frames per second; at lower setting, of course, image is not perceived as continuous. Nowadays, fluoroscopy can be acquired, sent to the PACS and stored, to be reviewed on the currently available high-resolution monitors. At the same time, alternatively, fluoroscopy can be stored and reviewed on dedicated digital recorders (Figure 2.4).

2.4 FLUOROSCOPY VERSUS RADIOGRAPHY

A controversial argument among radiologists dedicated to gastrointestinal tract imaging is regarding the various advantages and disadvantages of fluoroscopy and radiography. Radiography yields higher resolution and greater anatomic detail than fluoroscopic images. Cineradiography allows a better study of motion but yields lower resolution than static images and is, however, associated with larger radiation doses to the patient. Fluoroscopy studies, either analogically and digitally acquired, have the great advantage that they can be viewed in forward or reverse, and also in slow motion; the stop-frame images obtained through fluoroscopy have much lower resolution than digital radiographs. This argument about fluoroscopy versus radiography is still very much going on today, especially for the study of the pharynx; why some think that the analysis of function should have more emphasis, some others give more importance to the assessment of structural abnormalities, at the expense of the dynamical, functional analysis. Good news is that modern flat panel fluoroscopes produce better, improved fluoroscopic images that allow for a dynamical study of motion, even though static digital images yield a little lower resolution than conventional films (Figure 2.5). The possibility we have right now to acquire and store fluoroscopy images, cine-sequences that can be played over and over again for careful interpretation, is the actual founding principle of this book and the beginning of a new era for morphodynamic imaging (Figure 2.6).

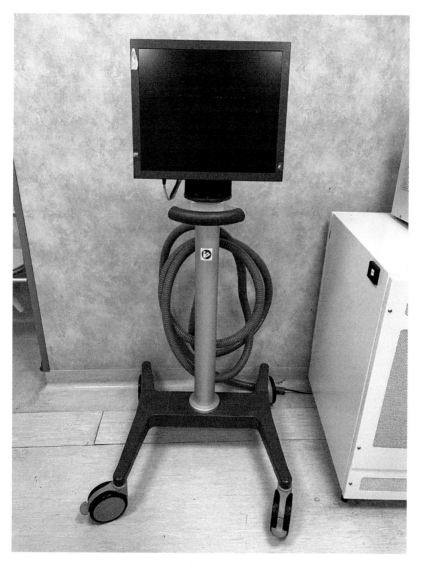

FIGURE 2.5   Digital fluoroscopic monitor.

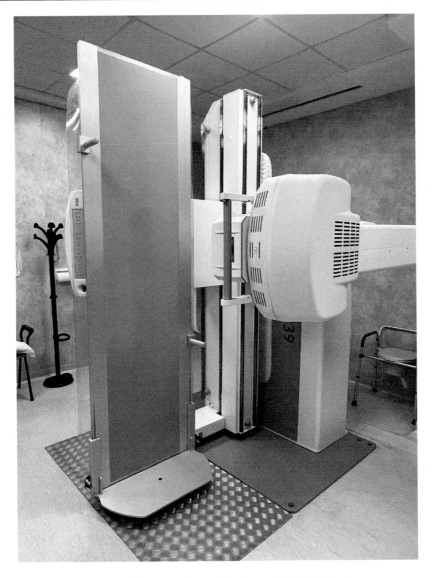

FIGURE 2.6   A radiology cabinet complete with tube and digital detector.

2.5 FURTHER READING

Aaddad NG, Fleischer DE. Neoplasms of the esophagus. In: Castell DO, editor. *The esophagus*. 2nd ed. Boston: Little, Brown; 1995. p. 269–91.

Agha FP, Lee HH, Nostant TT. Herpetic esophagitis: a diagnostic challenge in immunocompromised patients. *Am J Gastroenterol*. 1986;81:246–53.

Anbari MM, Laufer I. Development of gastrointestinal radiology. In: Gore RM, Levine MS, Laufer I, editors. *Textbook of gastrointestinal radiology*. Philadelphia: WB Saunders, Philadelphia; 1994. p. 2–16.

Andren L, Theander G. Roentgenographic appearances of esophageal moniliasis. *Acta Radiol.* 1956;46:571–4.

Attwood SE, Smyrk TC, DeMeester TR, Jones JB. Esophageal eosinophilia with dysphagia: a distinct clinicopathologic syndrome. *Dig Dis Sci.* 1993;38:109–16.

Bachem C, Gunther H. Barium sulfate as a shadow-forming contrast agent in roentgenologic examinations. *Zeitschrift f Röntg.* 1910;12:369–76.

Balfe DM, Koehler RE, Setzen M, Weyman PJ, Baron RL, Oqura JH. Barium examination of the esophagus after total laryngectomy. *Radiology.* 1982;143:501.

Bosch A, Frias Z, Caldwell WL. Adenocarcinoma of the esophagus. *Cancer.* 1979;43:1557–61.

Cannon WB. The passage of different food stuffs from the stomach and through the small intestines. *Am J Physiol.* 1904;12:387–418.

Carman RD, Miller A. *The roentgen diagnosis of diseases of the alimentary tract*. Philadelphia: WB Saunders; 1917.

Chen YM, Gelfand DW, Ott DJ, Wu WC. Barrett esophagus as an extension of severe esophagitis: analysis of radiologic signs in 29 cases. *AJR.* 1985;145:275–81.

Chen YM, Ott DJ, Gelfand DW, Munitz HA. Multiphasic examination of the esophagogastric region for strictures, rings, and hiatal hernia: evaluation of the individual techniques. *Gastrointest Radiol.* 1985;10:311.

Creteur V, Thoeni RF, Federle MP, et al. The role of single and double-contrast radiography in the diagnosis of reflux esophagitis. *Radiology.* 1983;147:71–5.

Croese J, Fairley SK, Masson JW, et al. Clinical and endoscopic features of eosinophilic esophagitis in adults. *Gastrointest Endosc.* 2003;58:516–22.

Curtis DJ. Laryngeal dynamics. *Crit Rev Diagn Imaging.* 1982;19:29–80.

Curtis DJ, Braham SL, Karr S, Holborow GS, Worman D. Identification of unopposed intact muscle pair actions affecting swallowing: potential for rehabilitation. *Dysphagia.* 1988;3:57–64.

Dantas RO, Dodds WJ, Massey BT, Kern MK. The effect of high- vs low-density barium preparations on the quantitative features of swallowing. *AJR.* 1989;153:1191.

Dantas RO, Kern MK, Massey BT, et al. Effect of swallowed bolus variables on oral and pharyngeal phases of swallowing. *Am J Physiol.* 1990;258:675–81.

Depew WT, Prentice RS, Beck IT, Blakeman JM, DaCosta LR. Herpes simplex ulcerative esophagitis in a healthy subject. *Am J Gastroenterol.* 1977;68:381–5.

Deshmukh M, Shah R, McCallum RW. Experience with herpes esophagitis in otherwise healthy patients. *Am J Gastroenterol.* 1984;79:173–6.

Dibble C, Levine MS, Rubesin SE, Laufer I, Katzka DA. Detection of reflux esophagitis on double-contrast esophagrams and endoscopy using the histologic findings as the gold standard. *Abdom Imaging.* 2004;29:421–5.

DiSantis DJ, Balfe DM, Koehler RE, et al. Barium examination of the pharynx after vertical hemilaryngectomy. *AJR.* 1983;141:335–9.

Dodds WJ, Man KM, Cook IJ, Kahrilas PJ, Stewart ET, Kern MK. Influence of bolus volume on swallow-induced hyoid movement in normal subjects. *AJR.* 1988;150:1307.

Dodds WJ, Stewart ET, Logemann JA. Physiology and radiology of the normal oral and pharyngeal phases of swallowing. *AJR.* 1990;154:953.

Dodds WJ, Taylor AJ, Stewart ET, Kern MK, Logemann JA, Cook IJ. Tipper and dipper types of oral swallows. *AJR.* 1989;153:1197.

Doty RW, Bosma JF. An electromyographic analysis of reflex deglutition. *J Neurophysiol.* 1956;19:44–60.

DuBrul EL. *Sicher's oral anatomy*. 7th ed. St. Louis: CV Mosby; 1980. p. 319.

Ekberg O, Feinberg MJ. Altered swallowing function in elderly patients without dysphagia: radiologic findings in 56 cases. *AJR.* 1991;156:1181.

Eras P, Goldstein MJ, Sherlock P. Candida infection of the gastrointestinal tract. *Medicine.* 1972;51:369–79.

Fox VL, Nurko S, Furuta GT. Eosinophilic esophagitis: it's not just kid's stuff. *Gastrointest Endosc.* 2002;56:260–70.

Gelfand DW. High density, low viscosity barium for fine mucosal detail on double-contrast upper gastrointestinal examinations. *AJR.* 1970;130:831–3.

Gilchrist AM, Levine MS, Carr RF, et al. Barrett's esophagus: diagnosis by double-contrast esophagography. *AJR.* 1988;150:97–102.

Graziani L, De Nigris E, Pesaresi A, Baldelli S, Dini L, Montesi A. Reflux esophagitis: radiologic-endoscopic correlation in 29 symptomatic cases. *Gastrointest Radiol.* 1983;1:1–6.

Gupta S, Levine MS, Rubesin SE, Katzka DA, Laufer I. Usefulness of barium studies for differentiating benign and malignant strictures of the esophagus. *AJR.* 2003;180:737–44.

Hewson EG, Richter JE. Gastroesophageal reflux disease. In: Gelfand DW, Richter JE, editors. *Dysphagia: diagnosis and treatment.* New York: Igaku-Shoin; 1989. p. 221–55.

Hsu WC, Levine MS, Rubesin SE. Overlap phenomenon: a potential pitfall in the radiographic detection of lower esophageal rings. *AJR.* 2003;180:745–7.

Jones B. *Normal and abnormal swallowing.* 2nd ed. Berlin: Springer; 2002.

Kodsi BE, Wickremesinghe PC, Kozinn PJ, Iswara K, Goldberg PK. Candida esophagitis: a prospective study of 27 cases. *Gastroenterology.* 1976;71:715–19.

Koehler RE, Weyman PJ, Oakley HF. Single- and double-contrast techniques in esophagitis. *AJR.* 1980;135:15–19.

Laufer I. *Double contrast gastrointestinal radiology with endoscopic correlation.* Philadelphia: WB Saunders; 1977.

Laufer I, Hamilton J, Mullens JE. Demonstration of superficial gastric erosions by double contrast radiology. *Gastroenterology.* 1975;68:387–91.

Leonard CL. The radiography of the stomach and intestines. *AJR.* 1913;1:1–42.

Levine MS. Gastroesophageal reflux disease. In: Gore RM, Levine MS, editors. *Textbook of gastrointestinal radiology.* 4th ed. Philadelphia: Elsevier; 2015. p. 291–311.

Levine MS. Infectious esophagitis. In: Gore RM, Levine MS, editors. *Textbook of gastrointestinal radiology.* 4th ed. Philadelphia: Elsevier; 2015. p. 312–25.

Levine MS, Ahmad NA, Rubesin SE. Elevated Z line: a new sign of Barrett's esophagus on double-contrast barium esophagograms. *Clin Imaging.* 2015;39:1103–4.

Levine MS, Caroline D, Thompson JJ, Kressel HY, Laufer I, Herlinger H. Adenocarcinoma of the esophagus: relationship to Barrett mucosa. *Radiology.* 1984;150:305–9.

Levine MS, Chu P, Furth EE, Rubesin SE, Laufer I, Herlinger H. Carcinoma of the esophagus and esophagogastric junction: sensitivity of radiographic diagnosis. *AJR.* 1997;168:1423–6.

Levine MS, Halvorsen RA. Esophageal carcinoma. In: Gore RM, Levine MS, editors. *Textbook of gastrointestinal radiology.* 4th ed. Philadelphia: Elsevier; 2015. p. 366–93.

Levine MS, Kressel HY, Caroline DF, Laufer I, Herlinger H, Thompson JJ. Barrett esophagus: reticular pattern of the mucosa. *Radiology.* 1983;147:663–7.

Levine MS, Laufer I. The gastrointestinal tract: dos and don'ts of digital imaging. *Radiology.* 1998;207:311.

Levine MS, Laufer I, Kressel HY, Friedman HM. Herpes esophagitis. *AJR.* 1981;136:863–6.

Levine MS, Loercher G, Katzka DA, Herlinger H, Rubesin SE, Laufer I. Giant, human immunodeficiency virus-related ulcers in the esophagus. *Radiology.* 1991;180:323–6.

Levine MS, Loevner LA, Saul SH, Rubesin SE, Herlinger H, Laufer I. Herpes esophagitis: sensitivity of double-contrast esophagography. *AJR.* 1988;151:57–62.

Levine MS, Macones AJ, Laufer I. Candida esophagitis: accuracy of radiographic diagnosis. *Radiology.* 1985;154:581–7.

Levine MS, Ott DJ, Laufer I. Barium studies: single and double contrast. In: Gore RM, Levine MS, editors. *Textbook of gastrointestinal radiology.* 4th ed. Philadelphia: Elsevier; 2015. p. 23–40.

Levine MS, Rubesin SE, Herlinger H, Laufer I. Double-contrast upper gastrointestinal examination: technique and interpretation. *Radiology*. 1988;168:593–602.

Levine MS, Rubesin SE, Laufer I. Barium esophagography: a study for all seasons. *Clin Gastroenterol Hepatol*. 2008;6:11–25.

Levine MS, Woldenberg R, Herlinger H, Laufer I. Opportunistic esophagitis in AIDS: radiographic diagnosis. *Radiology*. 1977;165:815–20.

Livstone EM, Skinner DB. Tumors of the esophagus. In: Berk JE, editor. *Bockus gastroenterology*. 4th ed. Philadelphia: Saunders; 1985. p. 818–50.

Logemann JA. *Evaluation and treatment of swallowing disorders*. Austin, TX: Pro-Ed; 1983.

Markowitz JE, Liacouras CA. Eosinophilic esophagitis. *Gastroenterol Clin North Am*. 2003; 32:949–66.

Marks RD, Richter JE. Peptic strictures of the esophagus. *Am J Gastroenterol*. 1993;88:1160–73.

Millan MS, Bourdages R, Beck IT, Da Costa LR. Transition from diffuse esophageal spasm to achalasia. *J Clin Gastroenterol*. 1979;1:107–17.

Missakian MM, Carlson HC, Andersen HA. The roentgenologic features of the columnar epithelial-lined lower esophagus. *AJR*. 1967;99:212–17.

Nickoloff EL. AAPM/RSNA physics tutorial for residents: physics of flat-panel fluoroscopy systems survey of modern fluoroscopy imaging: flat-panel detectors versus image intensifiers and more. *RadioGraphics*. 2011;31:591–602.

Nickoloff EL, Lu, ZF, Newhouse JH, Van Heertum R. *RSNA physics modules*. Fluoroscopy. www.rsna.org/Physics-Modules.

Niemeyer JH, Balfe DM, Hayden RE. Neck evaluation with barium-enhanced radiographs and CT scans after supraglottic subtotal laryngectomy. *Radiology*. 1987;162:493–8.

Ott DJ, Chen YM, Hewson EG, et al. Esophageal motility: assessment with synchronous video tape fluoroscopy and manometry. *Radiology*. 1989;173:419–22.

Ott DJ, Chen YM, Wu WC, Gelfand DW. Endoscopic sensitivity in the detection of esophageal strictures. *J Clin Gastroenterol*. 1985;7:121.

Ott DJ, Chen YM, Wu WC, Gelfand DW, Munitz HA. Radiographic and endoscopic sensitivity in detecting lower esophageal mucosal ring. *AJR*. 1986;147:261.

Ott DJ, Gelfand DW, Lane TG, et al. Radiologic detection and spectrum of appearances of peptic esophageal strictures. *J Clin Gastroenterol*. 1982;4:11.

Ott DJ, Gelfand DW, Wu WC. Reflux esophagitis: radiographic and endoscopic correlation. *Radiology*. 1979;130:583–8.

Ott DJ, Levine MS. Motility disorders of the esophagus. In: Gore RM, Levine MS, editors. *Textbook of gastrointestinal radiology*. 4th ed. Philadelphia: Elsevier; 2015. p. 279–90.

Ott DJ, Wu WC, Gelfand DW. Reflux esophagitis revisited: prospective analysis of radiologic accuracy. *Gastrointest Radioll*. 1981;6:1–7.

Owensby LC, Stammer JL. Esophagitis associated with herpes simplex infection in an immunocompetent host. *Gastroenterology*. 1978;74:1305–6.

Pearce J, Dagradi A. Acute ulceration of the esophagus with associated intranuclear inclusion bodies. *Arch Pathol*. 1943;35:889–97.

Prabhakar A, Levine MS, Rubesin SE, Laufer I, Katzka D. Relationship between diffuse esophageal spasm and lower esophageal sphincter dysfunction on barium studies and manometry in 14 patients. *AJR*. 2004;183:409–13.

Rabeneck L, Popovic M, Gartner S, et al. Acute HIV infection presenting with painful swallowing and esophageal ulcers. *JAMA*. 1990;263:2318–22.

Raphael HA, Ellis FH, Dockerty MB. Primary adenocarcinoma of the esophagus: 18-year review and review of literature. *Ann Surg*. 1966;164:785–96.

Rauschecker AM, Levine MS, Whitson MJ, et al. Esophageal lichen planus: clinical and radiographic findings in eight patients. *AJR*. 2017;208:1–6.

Robbins AH, Hermos JA, Schimmel EM, Friedlander DM, Messian RA. The columnar-lined esophagus–analysis of 26 cases. *Radiology*. 1977;123:1–7.

Rubesin SE, Glick SN. The tailored double-contrast pharyngogram. *CRC Crit Rev Diagn Imaging*. 1988;28:133–79.

Rubesin SE, Jessurun J, Robertson D, Jones B, Bosma JF, Donner MW. Lines of the pharynx. *RadioGraphics*. 1987;7:217–37.

Rubesin SE, Laufer I. Pictorial review: principles of double-contrast pharyngography. *Dysphagia*. 1991;6:170–8.

Rumpel T. Visualization of esophagus of patient with dysphagia with bismuth. *Muench Med Wochenschr*. 1897;44:420.

Schueler BA. The AAPM/RSNA physics tutorial for residents: general overview of fluoroscopic imaging. *RadioGraphics*. 2000;20:1115–26.

Sheft DJ, Shrago G. Esophageal moniliasis: the spectrum of the disease. *JAMA*. 1970;213:1852.

Shirakabe H. *Double contrast studies of the stomach*. Stuttgart: Georg Thieme Verlag; 1972.

Shortsleeve MJ, Gauvin GP, Gardner RC, Greenberg MS. Herpetic esophagitis. *Radiology*. 1981;141:611–17.

Skucas J. Contrast media. In: Gore RM, Levine MS, Laufer I, editors. *Textbook of gastrointestinal radiology*. Philadelphia: WB Saunders; 1994. p. 17–30.

Sor S, Levine MS, Kowalski TE, Laufer I, Rubesin SE, Herlinger H. Giant ulcers of the esophagus in patients with human immunodeficiency virus: clinical, radiographic, and pathologic findings. *Radiology*. 1995;194:447–51.

Thexton AJ, Crompton AW, German RZ. Electromyographic activity during the reflex pharyngeal swallow in the pig: doty and Bosma (1956) revisited. *J Appl Physiol*. 2007;102:587–600.

Thrift AP. The epidemic of oesophageal carcinoma: where are we now? *Cancer Epidemiol*. 2016;41:88–95.

Turnbull AD, Goodner JT. Primary adenocarcinoma of the esophagus. *Cancer*. 1968;22:915–18.

Vahey TN, Maglinte DD, Chernish SM. State-of-the-art barium examination in opportunistic esophagitis. *Dig Dis Sci*. 1986;31:1192–5.

Vitellas KM, Bennett WF, Bova JG, Johnson JC, Caldwell JH, Mayle JE. Idiopathic eosinophilic esophagitis. *Radiology*. 1993;186:789–93.

White SB, Levine MS, Rubesin SE, Spencer GS, Katzka DA, Laufer I. The small-caliber esophagus: radiographic sign of idiopathic eosinophilic esophagitis. *Radiology*. 2010;256:127–34.

Zimmerman SL, Levine MS, Rubesin SE, et al. Idiopathic eosinophilic esophagitis in adults: the ringed esophagus. *Radiology*. 2005;236:159–65.

Esophageal Anatomy and Physiology

3

Biondo Francesco Giuseppe, Russo Maurizio, Parente Emilio, and Pacifico Fabio

Contents

3.1 ANATOMY

The esophagus is a hollow muscular structure with two high-pressure zones, the upper and lower esophageal sphincters, which span 18–26 cm (Figure 3.1). It has a compressed oval shape in the axial plane, with the long axis extending laterally. The diameter is roughly 2 cm at rest and can reach up to 3 cm laterally when inflated with a meal bolus. Symptoms of dysphagia often appear when the lumen is constricted to less than 13 mm, improve when the lumen is more than 15 mm, and disappear completely when the lumen is greater than 18 mm. The esophagus, unlike the remainder of the gastrointestinal tract, lacks a genuine serosa. Mucosa, submucosa, muscularis propria, and adventitia are the four layers that make up the esophageal wall (Figure 3.2). A thin outer longitudinal layer and a broader inner circular layer split the muscularis propria. The esophagus is made up of striated muscle in the proximal third and smooth muscle in the distal third, with a moderate transition zone in between. On high-resolution esophageal manometry, this transition zone can be identified as a decrease or small break in peristalsis. The esophagus's motor

DOI: 10.1201/9781003320302-3

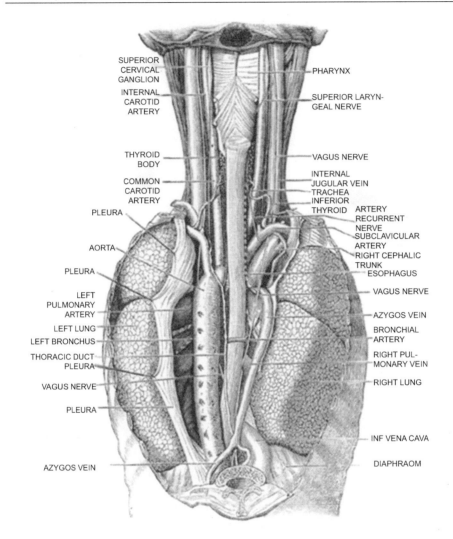

FIGURE 3.1 The esophagus and its course in the neck and thorax.

Source: Taken from *Gray's Anatomy*, 1918 Edition, public domain image.

activity is not rhythmic like the rest of the gastrointestinal tract's, and it is controlled by extrinsic and intrinsic innervations. Peristalsis is principally controlled in the proximal striated muscle by direct sequential vagal stimulation originating in the nucleus ambiguus. The peripheral enteric nervous system and central impulses from the dorsal motor nucleus work together to control peristalsis in the distal smooth muscle. Two nerve plexuses make up the peripheral enteric nervous system. The distal peristalsis is primarily coordinated by the myenteric plexus (Auerbach's plexus), which is located between the two muscular layers. The submucosal plexus (Meissner's plexus) is scarce in the esophagus and is primarily responsible for transmitting sensory information to the brain via vagal afferent neurons.

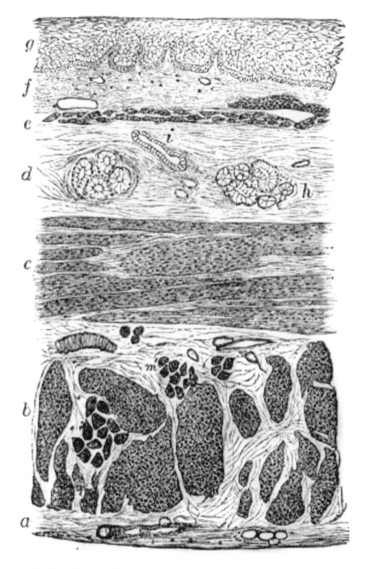

FIGURE 3.2 The four layers of the esophageal wall. Adventitia (a), Longitudinal (b) and Circular (c) Layers of the muscular propria, submucosa (d-f), Mucosa (g).

Source: Taken from *Gray's Anatomy*, 1918 Edition, public domain image.

Mucosal chemoreceptors and muscular mechanoreceptors can also send pain signals back to the somatosensory cortex via these same afferent neurons. Because of its large circulatory network, esophageal ischemia is relatively unusual. The vascular supply is variable, although branches from the inferior thyroid artery in the proximal third, the thoracic aorta in the middle third, and the left stomach artery in the distal third are the most common. Small tributaries discharge venous blood to the azygos and hemiazygos veins, which go to the superior vena cava in the thoracic cavity. The left gastric vein drains the distal esophagus. The development of distal esophageal varices is caused by retrograde flow through the left gastric vein in the presence of portal hypertension. Proximal esophageal varices, also known as downhill varices, occur infrequently and are mainly caused by obstruction of the superior vena cava. The esophagus is separated into three distinct segments based on topography: cervical, thoracic, and abdominal. The cervical esophagus begins where the inferior pharyngeal constrictor muscles join the cricopharyngeus muscle to form the upper esophageal sphincter (UES), a 1 cm high-pressure zone located at the level of C5–C6, and usually around 16 cm from the incisors. The UES is in a contracted position at rest to prevent air from entering and regurgitation from leaving the esophagus. Killian's triangle is a zone of scant musculature on the posterior wall immediately proximal to the UES. A Zenker's diverticulum might form in this location of relative muscular weakness. The most common cause of pharyngeal pressurization is poor UES opening due to cricopharyngeus muscle fibrosis, which results in a false diverticulum with only a mucosal and submucosal outpouching. The cervical esophagus is made entirely of striated muscle and extends about 5 cm along the cervical spine to the suprasternal notch. It is located between the carotid sheaths and the cervical vertebral bodies, posterior to the trachea and anterior to the trachea. Other common pathologies contributing to dysphagia can be observed in this area, including extrinsic compression from anterior cervical osteophytes and anterolateral outpouchings below the cricopharyngeus due to Killian-Jamieson diverticula, a congenital weakening of the esophagus wall. Rather than flowing straight down, the esophagus produces a modest reverse S shape when it enters the thoracic cavity, leaning to the left of the spinal column, then right, then left again. It creates several close relationships with the vasculature and airways as it descends, resulting in distinctive indentations that can be observed endoscopically. The aortic arch, which curves posteriorly and makes an impression on the left lateral wall of the esophagus, causes the initial indentation, which is around 23 cm from the incisors. Characteristic pulsations can often be seen on endoscopy to identify this. The left major bronchus passes anterior to the esophagus around 2 cm distal to this, causing a second depression. The esophagus lies below this, posterior to the left atrium of the heart, separated from it by a narrow pericardium. An enlarged left atrium might result in a third indentation. Any of these indentations, if accentuated, can cause dysphagia and are also places where pill esophagitis is more likely to occur. Dysphagia aortica is caused by the aorta compressing the esophagus, which usually occurs in the presence of a thoracic aortic aneurysm. Dysphagia lusoria is defined by a pencil-like indentation at T3–T4 above the aortic arch and is caused by an abnormal right subclavian artery, which affects 0.7% of the population. A short section of the esophagus (about 1 cm) reaches the abdomen as it departs the thoracic chamber through its own hiatus within the right crus of the diaphragm. The esophagus creates an indentation on the liver's left lobe's posterior surface. A second high-pressure zone, the lower esophageal sphincter (LES), marks the esophagus's distal end. The LES is made up of an asymmetrically thickened circular smooth muscle that is 2–4 cm long on average. The proximal border of the LES is difficult to discern endoscopically; however, the presence of a proportionally thickened muscular band can help. This area of the LES is sometimes referred to as the phrenic ampulla or vestibule on an esophagram. The LES and the crural diaphragm are two structures that make up the high-pressure zone at the esophagogastric junction (EGJ). The LES is made up of two muscular fibers called sling and clasp fibers (Figure 3.3). At the EGJ,

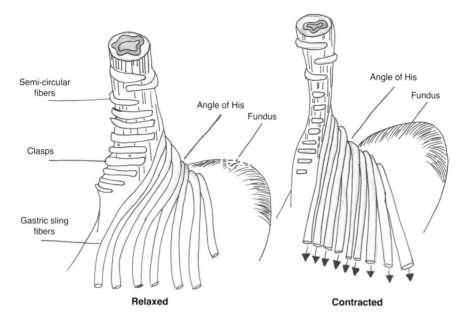

FIGURE 3.3 Sling and clasp fibers forming the LES. They cover the esophagus from the front, on the lesser curve side, and from the back. Sling fibers originate on the anterior gastric body, travel cephalad around the EGJ's larger curve side, and terminate on the posterior gastric body. Image art courtesy of Simona Borrelli.

the clasp fibers form an incomplete muscular ring. They cover the esophagus from the front, on the lesser curve side, and from the back. Sling fibers originate on the anterior gastric body, travel cephalad around the EGJ's larger curve side, and terminate on the posterior gastric body. The squamocolumnar junction is 1.5 cm proximal and 2 cm distal to the high-pressure zone. The phrenoesophageal ligament, which inserts circumferentially into the esophageal musculature, holds these two independent components of the EGJ in place. They can maintain a competent anti-reflux barrier by working together to constantly counterbalance a variable pressure gradient between the stomach and the esophagus and prevent excessive esophageal acid exposure. Now, the three esophageal sections, cervical, thoracic, and abdominal, can be further divided into smaller portions that come extremely useful from a radiologic and reporting point of view (Figure 3.4):

1. *Cervical portion* is the proximal section of the esophagus, its lower limit being the UES;
2. *Paratracheal portion* is the section coursing parallel to the trachea, its limits being the UES and the upper aspect of the aortic arch;
3. *Aortic portion* is the part of the esophagus compressed by the aortic arch;
4. *Aortobronchial portion* is the small section contained between the aortic and bronchial impressions of the esophagus;
5. *Bronchial portion* is the part of the esophagus compressed by the left bronchus;

6. *Cardiac portion* is the esophageal section compressed by the left atrium and posterior aspects of the heart;

7. *Epiphrenic section* is the slightly enlarged portion above the LES;

8. *Lower esophageal sphincter*, or lower pressure zone, is the portion of the esophagus between thorax and abdomen; and

9. *Abdominal portion* is the small section of the esophagus coursing into the abdomen and ending into the stomach at the EGJ.

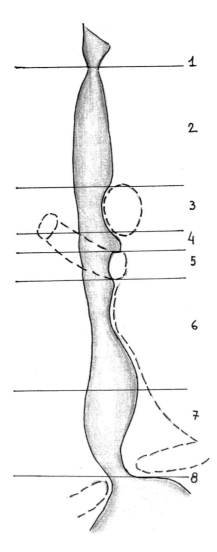

FIGURE 3.4 Esophageal Portions: 1. Cervical Portion; 2. Paratracheal Portion; 3. Aortic Portion; 4. Aortobronchial Portion; 5. Bronchial Portion; 6. Cardiac Portion; 7. Epiphrenic Section; 8. Lower Esophageal Sphincter, or Lower Pressure Zone. Image art courtesy of Simona Borrelli.

3.2 PHYSIOLOGY

3.2.1 Barrier Function

The esophageal epithelial barrier plays a critical role in protecting the underlying layers of the esophagus from harm caused by noxious chemicals. The pathophysiologic mechanisms of a range of disease conditions, including gastroesophageal reflux disease (GERD), Barrett's esophagus, and eosinophilic esophagitis, are influenced by changes in its structure and function. Pre-epithelial, epithelial, and post-epithelial are the three primary components of this barrier. A layer of water, bicarbonate, and mucin rests on the epithelium layer's surface as the pre-epithelial component. These three components are secreted by submucosal glands in the esophagus. The vagus appears to control, at least in part, the secretion of bicarbonate from the submucosal glands, which can be augmented when the esophagus is exposed to acid. Water and bicarbonate are also added to this layer by swallowed saliva. Water aids in the evacuation of acid present in the esophagus and preserves the underlying mucosa by diluting it further. This layer of protection is present, but it is not as strong as the one found in the stomach. The underlying layers of the esophagus would be more vulnerable to harm if the other two components of the esophageal barrier were missing. The epithelial component is made up of three layers of stratified squamous cells. The stratum corneum is the most superficial layer, consisting of flat cells that create a compact protective layer against luminal substances. The protein filaggrin, which helps to compact the cellular cytoskeleton, allows for this flat form. The presence of intercellular glycocalyx, which prevents material from moving between cells, adds to this protective barrier. The stratum spinosum is located beneath the stratum corneum. The presence of desmosomes, which connect adjacent cells and contribute to the barrier function of this layer, gives the cells in this layer a spiky look. This will be covered in greater depth further down. The stratum germinativum is the third and deepest layer. This layer's cells are the only ones capable of mitosis, and they're responsible for replacing cells in the deeper layers. The apical junction complex connects neighboring cells in the stratum corneum and stratum spinosum. This complex mediates paracellular transit, cell-cell signaling, and is the epithelial barrier's most durable component. It is made up of three major parts. The tight junction complex, which distinguishes the basolateral and apical cell surfaces and governs epithelial permeability, is the first and most apically positioned. A number of proteins form the tight junction complex, which joins neighboring intracellular cytoskeletons. Extracellular proteins such as claudin, occludin, and junctional adhesion molecules join neighboring cells. Zonulin is an intracellular protein that connects external proteins to actin in the cytoskeleton of the cell. The adherens junction is the second part of the apical junction complex. Vinculin, -catenin, and p 120-catenin are intracellular components that are joined to adjacent cells through the transmembrane protein epithelial-cadherin. The desmosome, the third and final component of the apical junction complex, offers mechanical support. Desmoglein and desmocolin are two extracellular proteins that connect to the intracellular cytoskeleton's keratin intermediate filaments via a cystoplasmic plaque. The third component of esophageal barrier function is the post-epithelial component.

The presence of an intercellular glyconjugate works as a buffer, neutralizing hydrogen ions that have escaped the other two components of the esophageal barrier. Finally, the esophagus mucosa's blood supply acts as a last barrier. It can remove hydrogen ions and metabolic waste and supply bicarbonate ions as a buffer against hydrogen ions. If injury occurs despite the esophageal barrier, the epithelium has two pathways for self-repair. The capacity of neighboring cells to migrate and replace necrotic ones is known as restitution. This is a quick procedure that can be completed in a matter of hours to give temporary repair. Epithelial cell replication can then take place over the next few days or weeks. Light microscopy, immunofluorescence methods, and transmission electron microscopy have all been used to investigate the structure of the esophageal epithelial barrier. These methods allow for the detection of dilated intercellular gaps, which are utilized as a marker of barrier structure and are an early sign of epithelial injury. For both in vivo and in vitro applications, methods to test esophageal barrier function have been developed. The measurement of mucosal impedance is used to determine barrier function in vivo. Endoscope probes that monitor impedance have been created in addition to typical 24-hour ambulatory pH and impedance probes. To determine mucosal impedance, both systems use a modified version of Ohm's law. This can be accomplished by applying a continuous voltage to two electrodes in close proximity to the mucosal surface. The current created as it passes through the mucosa from one electrode to the other is measured. $V/I=R$, where V is voltage, I is current, and R is resistance, which is comparable to impedance, is stated (Z). You may compute resistance or impedance by keeping the voltage constant and measuring current. Holding current constant while measuring voltage achieves the same result. When the impedance is low, more current can flow through the tissue. Alterations in impedance have been linked to esophageal barrier structural changes. Low impedance measures have been seen in erosive esophagitis, Barrett's esophagus, and eosinophilic esophagitis, among other diseases. Disruption of the aforementioned barrier systems causes changes in esophageal mucosal permeability, which can lead to a number of pathologic conditions. Both chemical injury and the inflammatory response associated with GERD alter the squamous epithelium's superficial luminal and basolateral cell layers. There is evidence that reflux can reduce claudin and epithelial cadherin expression, compromising the apical junction complex's function. There is a widening of intercellular gaps and basal cell hyperplasia in erosive esophagitis, in addition to increased intraepithelial lymphocytes within the mucosa. This means that the damage caused by reflux isn't just superficial; it also affects the underlying basal layer. As a result, continuing inflammatory alterations in the basal layer may contribute to the development of further harm. Barrett's esophagus, for example, is linked to abnormalities in esophageal barrier function. Intercellular spaces are also dilated in this situation, and there are changes in the expression and ratio of claudin subtypes within the apical junction complex. According to studies, the changes are linked to a change in tissue resistance, which could affect the epithelial tissue's response to additional injury. Finally, eosinophilic esophagitis is characterized by eosinophil infiltration of the esophageal epithelium. In this circumstance, several changes in barrier function have been seen. There have been reductions in zonulin, claudin, filaggrin, and intracellular space dilation. Desmosome malfunction has also been discovered, affecting the apical junction complex's structural integrity. These structural changes in the mucosal barrier are also linked to functional changes. The mucosal impedance of patients with eosinophilic esophagitis is lower than that of healthy controls. With the right treatment, mucosal impedance rises. Several esophageal disease states are marked by changes in barrier integrity and function. A better knowledge of the many pathways that contribute to this dysfunction could lead to the development of new treatments for these diseases.

3.2.2 Esophageal Motility

The esophagus and its sphincters have two basic functions: moving ingested boluses from the pharynx to the stomach and protecting the airways from unpleasant gastric contents. A peristaltic circular muscular contraction sweeps from the upper esophageal sphincter (UES) as it shuts to a relaxed lower esophageal sphincter to convey swallowed contents (LES). The peristaltic contraction's force fluctuates along the length of the esophagus, with the amplitude decreasing or disappearing in the striated-to-smooth muscle transition zone and increasing in the smooth muscular esophagus. Shortly after swallowing, the LES relaxes and stays relaxed until the peristaltic contraction reaches the esophagogastric junction (EGJ). The LES relaxes, reducing resistance to flow across the EGJ and enabling esophageal emptying into the stomach. Peristalsis in the striated muscular esophagus is fully controlled by somatic lower motor neurons that originate in the brainstem and proceed down the vagal nerves to the esophagus. These motor neurons fire in a craniocaudal sequence throughout the striated muscle esophagus, activating striated muscle motor units. We know this because swallow-induced peristalsis is eliminated by extremely proximal bilateral vagotomy, and electrical stimulation of the severed vagal nerve's caudal stump causes simultaneous circular muscular contraction along the striated muscle esophagus. Because swallow-induced peristalsis in the smooth muscle esophagus is inhibited by bilateral cervical vagotomy, it is initiated in the brainstem. The peristalsis program, on the other hand, is only peripheral in this region of the esophagus. A gradual circular muscular contraction is produced by electrical stimulation of the caudal vagal stump. The fact that peristalsis induced by esophageal distention (secondary peristalsis) is not removed by vagal disruption supports a peripheral mechanism programming peristalsis in this esophageal segment. Furthermore, when the smooth muscle part of the opossum esophagus is isolated from the CNS in vitro, it can induce peristalsis. For decades, the mechanism for peripheral programming of peristalsis in the smooth muscle esophagus has been a source of dispute and investigation. Simultaneous hyperpolarization of the circular smooth muscle membrane potential along the esophagus is produced by both vagal activation and swallowing. This hyperpolarization is followed by a transitory membrane depolarization, which is accompanied by a burst of smooth muscular action potentials that correlate to circular muscle contraction in both time and space. The duration of membrane hyperpolarization affects the timing of membrane depolarization, smooth muscle action potentials, and muscle contraction. By placing small strips of esophageal smooth muscle in a tissue bath and observing the contractile response to electrical stimuli that selectively activate myenteric neurons, previously known as nonadrenergic, noncholinergic nerves, the neuromuscular mechanisms underlying esophageal motor functions were studied. The circular smooth muscle contracts very little or not at all when these neurons are stimulated with trains of electrical pulses. There is a latency phase after the stimulus stops, followed by a delayed contraction known as the off-response. Muscular strips taken from the proximal smooth muscle esophagus have the shortest delay period, which increases as the smooth muscle segment lengthens. Vagal stimulation can also cause an off-response. During electrical stimulation that induces the off-response, electrophysiological recordings from circular smooth muscle cells demonstrate a hyperpolarization of the circular muscle membrane followed by a transitory depolarization that can be connected with action potentials. The duration of hyperpolarization and, as a result, the time of depolarization, increases in a linear fashion down the esophagus. As a result, it appears that the latency time is influenced by the length of hyperpolarization, which in turn influences the timing of depolarization. There is strong evidence that nitric oxide (NO) released in response to nerve stimulation influences the time and magnitude of the off-reaction. NO synthase (NOS) inhibitors shorten the off-latency response and reduce its amplitude. NOS inhibitors at their highest dosages practically totally eliminate the off-response and reveal a cholinergic contraction. As one could assume based on the findings of these research, the timing of swallow-induced peristalsis in the smooth muscle esophagus is influenced by NO. At all levels of the smooth muscle esophagus, NOS inhibitors reduce the duration between swallowing and the onset of peristalsis. The distal esophagus shortens the most, increasing the velocity of peristalsis to the point where the pressure waves are almost synchronous. Under these conditions, atropine, a muscarinic cholinergic antagonist, reduces the amplitude of esophageal contraction and somewhat lengthens the latency, but by the same amount along the smooth muscle esophagus. Furthermore, when individuals were administered intravenously recombinant human hemoglobin, which avidly binds NO, normal peristalsis was changed to motor patterns that resembled achalasia and esophageal spasm. These and other studies imply that NO is predominantly responsible for peristalsis timing in the smooth muscle esophagus, and that acetylcholine is primarily responsible for contraction power and, to a lesser extent, time. Swallowing causes esophageal shortening, which, like peristalsis, follows a craniocaudal pattern but occurs before the peristaltic circular muscle contraction. Peristalsis is caused by the activation of muscarinic cholinergic motor neurons, but unlike smooth muscle, it is controlled by vagal efferent fibers in the brainstem. Esophageal shortening is hypothesized to increase luminal diameter ahead of the bolus, lowering bolus transit resistance and thickening esophageal musculature to improve contraction force. The EGJ closes at rest due to tonic contraction of the lower esophageal sphincter (LES) muscles and crural diaphragm contraction. The length-tension characteristics of circular strips of muscle taken from the EGJ and adjacent esophagus and stomach of the opossum were first demonstrated by comparing the length-tension characteristics of circular strips of muscle taken from the EGJ and adjacent esophagus and stomach of the opossum. When muscle strips from all three locations were stretched, the EGJ muscle produced higher tone for the same amount of stretch, demonstrating that it creates tone at rest, indicating that it is a physiological sphincter. Because the LES muscle strip was isolated from the CNS, the mechanisms that generate tone must be internal to the muscle tissue. Tetrodotoxin, a sodium channel blocker that prevents neuronal action potentials, had no influence on LES tone in the opossum, implying that the majority, if not all, of the tone is myogenic. Since atropine lowers resting tone, NOS inhibitors can increase it, and vagal activity can modify LES tone in other species, including humans, there is evidence for some resting LES tone being neurogenic in vivo. Because calcium channel blockers do not completely eliminate LES tone, and extracellular calcium removal only partially decreases it, the LES generates intrinsic tone that is dependent on intracellular and extracellular calcium. According to some data, the LES muscle is toned because its free cytosolic calcium concentration is higher than that of adjacent esophageal or gastric muscle. There is additional evidence that the LES produces tone because it has a lower negative membrane potential than other esophageal smooth muscle. Whatever mechanisms are responsible for LES muscle's resting tone, its energy metabolism is separate from that of nearby esophageal smooth muscle. Aerobic mechanisms sustain LES muscular tone, but anaerobic conditions maintain phasic contractions in adjacent esophageal muscle. Furthermore, straining the LES muscle to generate tone increases oxygen consumption significantly, whereas stretching the neighboring esophageal circular smooth muscle produces little tone and no increase in oxygen consumption. Finally, the capacity of circular LES muscle to maintain contraction using substrates other than glucose differs significantly from that of adjacent esophageal muscle. The crural diaphragm contributes to the sphincter mechanism in the distal esophagus by contracting. At the level of the EGJ, it contributes to both resting and phasic pressure increases recorded in the typical high-pressure zone. The tonic contraction of the circular LES muscle is hypothesized to cause end-expiratory pressure at the EGJ. The crural diaphragm contraction is assumed to be the cause of increased pressure during inspiration. Because bilateral vagotomy eliminates the relaxation of the LES generated by swallowing, it is vagally mediated. The vagal efferent neurons that cause LES relaxation emerge from the brain stem and connect to myenteric neurons in the LES. They secrete acetylcholine, which stimulates secondary, inhibitory myenteric neurons that terminate in the LES smooth muscle. As a result, the LES relaxes. Hyperpolarization of the muscular membrane is the electrophysiological response associated with relaxation of the LES circular smooth muscle in response to swallowing, vagal activation, or stimulation of intrinsic myenteric neurons. NO is the major neurotransmitter that causes muscular hyperpolarization and relaxation in the LES. Exogenous nitric oxide promotes relaxation and hyperpolarization of the membrane potential of isolated LES circular muscle. Nerve-induced relaxation and hyperpolarization of the LES muscle are inhibited by NOS inhibitors. During intrinsic nerve stimulation, nitric oxide is released from LES tissue, and immunohistochemistry methods detect NOS in LES and esophageal myenteric neurons. A number of peptides found in myenteric LES neurons, such as VIP and CGRP, have been postulated as LES relaxation mediators. Electrical stimulation of myenteric neurons causes biphasic LES relaxation in isolated LES. During the stimulation, there is a fast and a sustained component. The fast component was suppressed by an antagonist of NOS and hemoglobin, while the sustained component was unaffected. VIP or CGRP inhibitors showed little effect on either component of relaxation, implying that they are unlikely mediators of LES relaxation.

3.3 FURTHER READING

Almeida T, Roizenblatt S, Tufik S. Afferent pain pathways: a neuroanatomical review. *Brain Res* 2004; 1000: 40–56.

Aziz Q, Rothwell J, Barlow J, et al. Esophageal myoelectric responses to magnetic stimulation of the human cortex and the extracranial vagus nerve. *Am J Physiol* 1994; 267 (Pt 1): 64. G827–35.

Bardan E, Xie P, Aslam M, Kern M, Shaker R. Disruption of primary and secondary esophageal peristalsis by afferent stimulation. *Am J Physiol Gastrointest Liver Physiol* 2000; 279: G255–61.

Bieger D. Neuropharmacologic correlates of deglutition: lessons from fictive swallowing. *Dysphagia* 1991; 6: 147.

Christensen J. Mechanisms of secondary esophageal peristalsis. *Am J Med* 1997; 103: 44S–6S.

Clouse R, Staiano A. Topography of the esophageal peristaltic pressure wave. *Am J Physiol* 1991; 261 (Pt 1): G677–84.

Clouse R, Staiano A, Bickston S, Cohn S. Characteristics of the propagating pressure wave in the esophagus. *Dig Dis Sci* 1996; 41: 2369–76.

Daniel E, Bardakjian B, Huizinga J, Diamant N. Relaxation oscillator and core conductor models are needed for understanding of GI electrical activities. *Am J Physiol* 1994; 266 (Pt 1): G339–49.

Dent J, Dodds W, Friedman R, et al. Mechanism of gastroesophageal reflux in recumbent asymptomatic human subjects. *J Clin Invest* 1980; 65: 256–67.

Diamant N. Physiology of esophageal motor function. *Gastroenterol Clin North Am* 1989; 18: 179–94.

Eslami M, Richards W, Sugarbaker D. Esophageal physiology. *Chest Surg Clin N Am* 1994; 4: 635–52.

Farré R, Fornari F, Blondeau K et al. Acid and weakly acidic solutions impair mucosal integrity of distal exposed and proximal non-exposed human oesophagus. *Gut* 2010; 59: 164–9.

Fass R. Sensory testing of the esophagus. *J Clin Gastroenterol* 2004; 38: 628–41.

Garrison D, Chandler M, Foreman R. Viscerosomatic convergence onto feline spinal neurons from esophagus, heart and somatic fields: effects of inflammation. *Pain* 1992; 49: 373–82.

Ghosh S, Janiak P, Fox M, Schwizer W, Hebbard G, Brasseur J. Physiology of the oesophageal transition zone in the presence of chronic bolus retention: studies using concurrent high resolution manometry and digital fluoroscopy. *Neurogastroenterol Motil* 2008; 20: 750–9.

Ghosh S, Janiak P, Schwizer W, Hebbard G, Brasseur J. Physiology of the esophageal pressure transition zone: separate contraction waves above and below. *Am J Physiol Gastrointest Liver Physiol* 2006; 290: G568–76.

Gidda J, Goyal R. Influence of successive vagal stimulations on contractions in esophageal smooth muscle of opossum. *J Clin Invest* 1983; 71: 1095–103.

Goyal R, Gidda J. Relation between electrical and mechanical activity in esophageal smooth muscle. *Am J Physiol* 1981; 240: G305–11.

Janssens J, De Wever I, Vantrappen G, Hellemans J. Peristalsis in smooth muscle esophagus after transection and bolus deviation. *Gastroenterology* 1976; 71: 1004–9.

Kahrilas P, Dodds W, Hogan W. Effect of peristaltic dysfunction on esophageal volume clearance. *Gastroenterology* 1988; 94: 73–80.

Kahrilas P, Ghosh S, Pandolfino J. Esophageal motility disorders in terms of pressure topography: the Chicago classification. *J Clin Gastroenterol* 2008; 42: 627–35.

Knowles C, Aziz Q. Visceral hypersensitivity in non-erosive reflux disease. *Gut* 2008; 57: 674–83.

Li M, Brasseur J, Dodds W. Analyses of normal and abnormal esophageal transport using computer simulations. *Am J Physiol* 1994; 266 (Pt 1): G525–43.

Long J, Orlando R. Esophageal submucosal glands: structure and function. *Am J Gastroenterol* 1999; 94: 2818–24.

Mayer E, Gebhart G. Basic and clinical aspects of visceral hyperalgesia. *Gastroenterology* 1994; 107: 271–93.

Meyer G, Gerhardt D, Castell D. Human esophageal response to rapid swallowing: muscle refractory period or neural inhibition? *Am J Physiol* 1981; 241: G129–36.

Miranda A, Nordstrom E, Mannem A, Smith C, Banerjee B, Sengupta J. The role of transient receptor potential vanilloid 1 in mechanical and chemical visceral hyperalgesia following experimental colitis. *Neuroscience* 2007; 148: 1021–32.

Nicosia M, Brasseur J, Liu J, Miller L. Local longitudinal muscle shortening of the human esophagus from high-frequency ultrasonography. *Am J Physiol Gastrointest Liver Physiol* 2001; 281: G1022–33.

Pandolfino J, Fox M, Bredenoord A, Kahrilas P. High-resolution manometry in clinical practice: utilizing pressure topography to classify oesophageal motility abnormalities. *Neurogastroenterol Motil* 2009; 21: 796–806.

Pandolfino J, Leslie E, Luger D, Mitchell B, Kwiatek M, Kahrilas P. The contractile deceleration point: an important physiologic landmark on oesophageal pressure topography. *Neurogastroenterol Motil* 2010; 22: 395–400, e90.

Pandolfino J, Shi G, Zhang Q, Kahrilas P. Absence of a deglutitive inhibition equivalent with secondary peristalsis. *Am J Physiol Gastrointest Liver Physiol* 2005; 288: G671–6.

Paterson W. Electrical correlates of peristaltic and nonperistaltic contractions in the opossum smooth muscle esophagus. *Gastroenterology* 1989; 97: 665–75.

Patterson L, Zheng H, Ward S, Berthoud H. Vanilloid receptor (VR1) expression in vagal afferent neurons innervating the gastrointestinal tract. *Cell Tissue Res* 2003; 311: 277–87.

Pouderoux P, Lin S, Kahrilas P. Timing, propagation, coordination, and effect of esophageal shortening during peristalsis. *Gastroenterology* 1997; 112: 1147–54.

Qin C, Chandler M, Foreman R. Esophagocardiac convergence onto thoracic spinal neurons: comparison of cervical and thoracic esophagus. *Brain Res* 2004; 1008: 193–7.

Qin C, Farber J, Foreman R. Gastrocardiac afferent convergence in upper thoracic spinal neurons: a central mechanism of postprandial angina pectoris. *J Pain* 2007; 8: 522–9.

Rattan S, Gidda J, Goyal R. Membrane potential and mechanical responses of the opossum esophagus to vagal stimulation and swallowing. *Gastroenterology* 1983; 85: 922–8.

Richter J, Wu W, Johns D, et al. Esophageal manometry in 95 healthy adult volunteers: variability of pressures with age and frequency of 'abnormal' contractions. *Dig Dis Sci* 1987; 32: 583–92.

Shi G, Pandolfino J, Joehl R, Brasseur J, Kahrilas P. Distinct patterns of oesophageal shortening during primary peristalsis, secondary peristalsis and transient lower oesophageal sphincter relaxation. *Neurogastroenterol Motil* 2002; 14: 505–12.

Sifrim D, Janssens J, Vantrappen G. A wave of inhibition precedes primary peristaltic contractions in the human esophagus. *Gastroenterology* 1992; 103: 876–82.

Sifrim D, Lefebvre R. Role of nitric oxide during swallow-induced esophageal shortening in cats. *Dig Dis Sci* 2001; 46: 822–30.

Sugarbaker D, Rattan S, Goyal R. Mechanical and electrical activity of esophageal smooth muscle during peristalsis. *Am J Physiol (Pt 1)* 1984; 246: G145–50.

Vanek A, Diamant N. Responses of the human esophagus to paired swallows. *Gastroenterology* 1987; 92: 643–50.

van Malenstein H, Farré R, Sifrim D. Esophageal dilated intercellular spaces (DIS) and nonerosive reflux disease. *Am J Gastroenterol* 2008; 103: 1021–8.

Weisbrodt N, Christensen J. Gradients of contractions in the opossum esophagus. *Gastroenterology* 1972; 62: 1159–66.

Woolf C. Evidence for a central component of post-injury pain hypersensitivity. *Nature* 1983; 306: 686–8.

Woolf C, Shortland P, Coggeshall R. Peripheral nerve injury triggers central sprouting of myelinated afferents. *Nature* 1992; 355: 75–8.

Yamato S, Spechler S, Goyal R. Role of nitric oxide in esophageal peristalsis in the opossum. *Gastroenterology* 1992; 103: 197–204.

Zhang X, Geboes K, Depoortere I, Tack J, Janssens J, Sifrim D. Effect of repeated cycles of acute esophagitis and healing on esophageal peristalsis, tone, and length. *Am J Physiol Gastrointest Liver Physiol* 2005; 288: G1339–46.

Pathophysiology of Achalasia

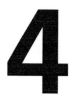

Giuseppe Fuggi, Francesca Russo, and Rocco Granata

Contents

4.1 INTRODUCTION

Primary achalasia is thought to be the outcome of a complicated interaction between numerous factors, according to literature. The main pathological feature of achalasia is the loss of ganglion cells both in the body of the esophagus and in patients genetically susceptible to the disease. Inflammatory and autoimmune responses, most likely triggered by viral infections, are strongly linked to the main pathological feature of achalasia: the loss of ganglion cells both in the body of the esophagus and in patients genetically susceptible to the disease. The loss of ganglion cells is significantly linked to collagen deposition and inflammation.

4.1.1 Infections

Despite the fact that the role of viral infections in the pathophysiology of achalasia and, in particular, in the induction of the loss of ganglion cells is still being debated, numerous

DOI: 10.1201/9781003320302-4

clinical studies have investigated the pathological potential of active neurotrophic and chronic latent infections, both viral and bacterial, in achalasia patients. There have been a number of proposed virus candidates (Table 4.1), including the herpes simplex virus (HSV), a neurotropic virus that has a preference for squamous epithelium, the John Cunningham virus (also known as "JC" virus), the bornavirus, the varicella zoster virus, measles, and the human papilloma virus. During latent infections, the persistent presence of the HSV-1 virus in neurons of the body of the esophagus and lower esophageal sphincter is thought to trigger neuronal destruction in patients with a genetic predisposition for achalasia. This would result in persistent immune activation, which would lead to ganglion cell loss. Another study linking viruses and achalasia is an epidemiological study and genotype-phenotype analysis conducted by Becker et al., in which it was demonstrated that patients with achalasia were frequently affected by viral infections, particularly varicella zoster virus infections, prior to the onset of the disease. The same study went even further, claiming that pregnancy may be a risk factor for the disease in HLA-DQ1 insertion carriers of the virus. Many pathology studies conducted on biopsy specimens from patients with idiopathic achalasia have revealed a probable association with herpes simplex virus type 1 (HSV-1). When looking for the presence of diverse virus strains in the myenteric plexus, the polymerase chain reaction has been extensively used. HSV-1 enters the body through the perioral and esophageal mucosa, which are its preferred entrance points. Furthermore, herpes viruses have a significant affinity for nerve fibers, and after a primary exposure, the viruses can persist in a latent form in neuronal nuclei for up to a year after the initial exposure. While it is well known that T cells respond particularly to HSV-1 antigens, it has been found that achalasia patients have a much greater rate of oligoclonal CD3+/CD8+ lymphocytic infiltrates in the lower epididymis when compared with healthy controls. Given that not all patients with viral infections acquire achalasia, it has been hypothesized that certain genetic alterations affecting the immune system may be responsible for the development of this disease vulnerability.

TABLE 4.1   Viruses Suspect of Involvement in the Pathogenesis of Achalasia.

HSV (HSV-1 in particular)
HPV
John Cunningham Virus (JCV)
Bornavirus
Measles
VZV

The presence of a chronic viral infection may result in an abnormal immunological response, which, when combined with an adequate genetic and environmental background, may facilitate the loss of esophageal neurons. The myenteric plexus of patients with achalasia has been demonstrated to be infiltrated with CD3+CD45RO+ T cells, primarily CD8+ T cytotoxic lymphocytes, which display activation markers, providing support for this hypothesis.

4.1.2 Ganglion Cell Loss

The enteric nervous system, which includes the esophagus, is found throughout the gastrointestinal tract. The myenteric plexus is made up of postganglionic neurons that differentiate into excitatory cholinergic neurons and inhibitory nitrergic neurons and is located between the circular and longitudinal smooth muscle layers of the gut. The inhibitory neurons emit the free radical NO and the neurotransmitter/anti-inflammatory cytokine VIP, while the excitatory neurons release acetylcholine; this synchronized release creates the balance of relaxation and contraction required for appropriate esophageal peristalsis. Achalasia is thought to be caused by a decrease in Cajal interstitial cells, as well as a selective loss of inhibitory ganglia in the myenteric plexus of the esophagus, which is linked to a decrease in NO and VIP. In a benzyldimethyltetradecylammonium chloride-induced amyenteric rat model and human tissues, these pathophysiological and morphologic aspects have been established. Furthermore, in experimental animal systems, nitrergic neurons were shown to mediate esophageal neuromuscular activities such as LES relaxation and proper peristalsis. Animal research have also revealed the genetic roots of achalasia for the first time. Mice with a disruption of the neuronal NO synthase 1 gene (nNOS-/-) had significantly increased hypertensive LES and, as a result, significantly impaired relaxation, which progressed to achalasia-like LES dysfunction and gastroparesis; these findings contrast with the hypotensive LES seen in W/Wv mice, which lack the interstitial cells of Cajal as a relaxation intermediary. NO innervation in the myenteric plexus of patients with achalasia has also been found to be considerably reduced or nonexistent in human investigations. Immunohistochemical examinations of biopsies from achalasia patients who had surgery revealed considerably lower levels of VIP, nNOS, neural proteins, S-100, substance P, and protein gene product 9.5 (PGP9.5) than in healthy people. As a result, decreased NO and VIP production may play a role in the pathogenesis of achalasia and may be genetic components as well as therapeutic targets. The esophageal myenteric immune-mediated response and inflammatory state, accompanied by T cell infiltration, are underlying pathogenic mechanisms in the early stages of achalasia, driven by an unknown etiologic source. With little early ganglion cell loss or only mild to severe fibrosis in the smooth muscle layer, this pathologic state can produce neuritis and ganglionitis. Transthyretin (TTR) is a serum and cerebrospinal fluid carrier of the thyroid hormone thyroxine (T4) and a retinol-binding protein that is associated with familial amyloid polyneuropathy, and its observed upregulation corroborates with the subsequent neural degeneration observed in patients, according to a proteomic analysis of serum from patients with achalasia and healthy individuals. Furthermore, elevated deposits of the complement complex C5b-C9 and IgM within or proximal to ganglion cells of the myenteric plexus have been found in several studies of achalasia patients. Loss of VIP- and NO-secreting neurons causes an imbalance that can result in irreversible esophageal motor impairment. Furthermore, the classic subtype of achalasia would result from the progressive death of myenteric ganglion cells and the formation of neural fibrosis. Hypertrophy and neuronal fibrosis accompany the illness progression, in addition to the death of inhibitory ganglionic cells (owing to the extensive inflammatory infiltrates and autoimmune). Neuronal autoantibodies are seen in the majority of reports of pathogenic findings in human instances. These autoimmune components have been proven to contribute directly to myenteric plexus damage. Bruley des Varannes et al., for example, have shown that serum from individuals with achalasia, but not from patients with GERD, can cause phenotypic and functional alterations in myenteric neurons that mimic illness symptoms, proving that autoantibodies are not an epiphenomenon. The potential causes of ganglion cell loss are summarized in Table 4.2.

TABLE 4.2   Causes of Ganglion Cell Loss.

Potential genetic disruptions
Autoimmune neuritis
Autoimmune ganglionitis
Decreased NO and VIP production
Decrease of Cajal cells
Loss of myenteric inhibitory ganglia

4.1.3 Autoimmunity

Anti-myenteric antibodies in the circulation and inflammatory T cell infiltrates in the myenteric plexus, as well as statistical connections between the disease and specific HLA class II antigens, support the postulated autoimmune origin of achalasia. Autoimmune disorders frequently occur in conjunction with one another, either in a single person or within a family. An autoimmune component has been hypothesized as part of the achalasia etiology. Patients with achalasia are 3.6 times more likely to have autoimmune diseases (Table 4.3), according to findings from a recent study and numerous case reports, including uveitis (RR = 259), Sjögren's syndrome (RR = 37), systemic lupus erythematosus (RR = 43), type I diabetes (RR = 5.4), hypothyroidism (RR = 8.5), and rheumatoid arthritis (RR = 2.4). Surprisingly, a younger community of achalasia patients was shown to have a higher prevalence of autoimmune comorbidities (RR = 3.3) than an older population of achalasia patients. Finally, some patients with achalasia have responded to immunosuppressive medicines, supporting the theory that the condition is autoimmune in nature. Achalasia's etiology is most likely complex, involving genetic and immune-related variables, perhaps both pathogen/environmental and host-derived. An etiological profile like this could set off potentially harmful autoimmune processes or persistent inflammation.

TABLE 4.3   Associations with Autoimmunity.

Uveitis
Sjögren's syndrome
Systemic lupus erythematosus
Type I diabetes
Hypothyroidism
Rheumatoid arthritis

4.1.4 Inflammation

Inflammatory infiltrates of various strength surrounding myenteric neurons have also been discovered in the esophageal tissues of individuals with achalasia, in contrast to the non-infiltrate results of control groups with normal myenteric plexus. CD3+, CD4+, CD25+, and CD8+ T lymphocytes, as well as CD20+ B lymphocytes and eosinophilic granulocytes, predominated in all sick tissues, with sporadic plasma and mast cells detected along the nerve fascicles and around the ganglion cells. Furthermore, in tissues with advanced stage illness (> ten-year symptom history), T and B inflammatory infiltrates predominated. C4B5, C3, cyclin-dependent kinase 5, and 2-macroglobulin are upregulated in achalasia patients compared to controls, validating the idea of immune-mediated response and/or brain degeneration components of disease pathogenesis. Furthermore, the complement complex C5b-C9 (membrane assault complex) and IgM are deposited within or at the ganglion cells of the myenteric plexus in another investigation of achalasia patients. In achalasia patients, extracellular matrix turnover, as well as various CD4+ T cell subsets and cytokines, has been seen. In LES from patients with achalasia, a significant increase in the expression of matrix metalloproteinase-9 (MMP-9, commonly known as 92 kDa gelatinase) and its tissue inhibitor, TIMP1, was identified when compared to controls. In patients with achalasia, several tissue and circulating CD4+ T cell subsets have also been identified. Interleukin-22 (IL-22) expression has been found to be upregulated in achalasia patients' tissue (particularly the myenteric plexus) and circulating cells. IL-22 is a member of the IL-10 family of proteins that functions as an initiator of the innate immune response against pathogens in gut epithelium and respiratory cells, as well as a modulator of tissue repair and regeneration processes and a regulator of antibody formation. Th22 and Th17 are two subgroups of T helper (Th) cells that produce IL-22. In response to TNF- and IL-6 signals, Th22 cells develop from naive T cells and synthesize and secrete IL-26, IL-13, and IL-22; IL-26 is involved in cellular proliferation and survival, antimicrobial peptide production, epithelial renewal, and immunity. The Th17 subset produces the cytokine IL-17A, which is a critical mediator of auto-inflammatory disorders. IL-17A stimulates T cells, increases the production of autoantibodies and inflammatory cytokines (TNF-, IL-1, IL-6, IL-8, IL-17, IL-22, etc.) and chemokines (CCL2, CCL7, CCL20, CXCL1, CXCL5), activates innate immune cells, and enhances B cell functions in both physiological and pathological conditions. Patients with achalasia have a higher frequency of IL-17A-secreting cells in their peripheral cells and myenteric plexus of esophageal tissue than controls. Interferon-gamma (IFN-) is another essential cytokine that may have a role in achalasia pathophysiology. IFN- controls numerous immunological and inflammatory responses and is produced by activated T cells and natural killer cells (NKs). This cytokine induces macrophages to ingest and destroy germs by potentiating the effects of type I IFNs, recruiting leukocytes to infected tissue to potentiate beneficial inflammation, and recruiting leukocytes to infected tissue to potentiate beneficial inflammation. Th1 cells also have a role in controlling the Th2 response by releasing IFN-. Because IFN- is so important in immune response modulation, abnormal regulation of its production might lead to autoimmune disorders. IFN- also inhibits collagen formation while promoting the production of chemokines such as CXCR3, CXCL9, CXCL10, and CXCL11. Achalasia patients had a significantly higher percentage of circulating and tissue IFN-+/CD4+ T cells than controls, according to studies. In tissue from achalasia patients, increased expression of IL-1, IL-2, and TNF- has also been identified when compared to controls. In patients with achalasia, several cytokines with dual anti-inflammatory/pro-fibrogenic activities have been studied. TGF-1 regulates cellular growth, proliferation, differentiation, negative regulation of inflammation, collagen synthesis, and apoptosis under normal physiologic conditions; patients with achalasia have significantly higher TGF-1+ cell expression in the myenteric plexus of esophageal biopsies than controls. IL-4 is an anti-inflammatory cytokine that regulates B cell proliferation and differentiation, suppresses apoptosis, and inhibits the manufacture of numerous key cytokines (IL-1, TNF-, IL-6, IL-17A, and others). Th2 cells are the main producers of IL-4, which is essential for the initiation and maintenance of fibrosis. The IL-4-expressing CD4+ Th2 subset is defined by IL-4, IL-5, IL-9, and IL-13 production and functions in type 2 immunity for fighting infectious disease, which includes toxin neutralization, metabolic homeostasis, wound healing, tissue regeneration, and the production and deposition of fibrosis-enhancing collagen; in addition, these cells suppress autoimmune disease mediated by Th1 cells. Achalasia patients had a much higher circulating and tissue IL-4+ cell percentage than controls, according to studies. IL-13 has comparable effects to IL-4, but it also regulates the type I collagen gene, which plays a role in fibrosis. It has a similar expression pattern to IL-4 in people with achalasia. T regulatory cells, also known as Tregs, are a subset of immune "regulatory cells" that have unique capabilities that allow them to impose cell extrinsic immunosuppression and tolerance to both self and foreign antigens. Tregs minimize tissue damage and autoimmunity by modulating the natural course of protective immune responses. They also suppress immune responses by generating granzymes and perforins, depleting IL-2, secreting suppressor molecules like IL-19 and TGF-1, and reducing the functions of antigen presentation cells (APCs), which would otherwise trigger anergy or apoptosis in effector T cells. Tregs play a vital function in tissue healing and homeostasis as a result. In the myenteric plexus of esophageal tissue, patients with achalasia had a greater Treg frequency than controls. Nonetheless, Sodikoff et al. reported that Foxp3 (a Treg-specific marker) was not detectable in their cohort's achalasia biopsies, in contrast to our findings, which showed a higher percentage of CD25+/Foxp3+ cells in esophageal smooth muscle tissue from patients with type III achalasia, followed by types I and II, when compared to controls. Different approaches utilized to conserve the samples prior to inspection or to perform the immunohistochemical evaluation could explain the discrepancies, or the findings could indicate significant changes in disease evolution between the two cohorts. In addition to Tregs, a newly identified population of regulatory B cells (dubbed Bregs) has been shown to contribute to immunosuppression, not only in autoimmune diseases but also in inflammatory and organ/tissue transplant conditions; regardless, the effects are direct and occur via Treg function enhancement. In an IL-10-dependent way, this CD19+CD24hiCD38hi immature/transitional T1 B cell subpopulation reduces Th1 cell development. Surprisingly, biopsies of the myenteric plexus taken from achalasia patients revealed a larger number of IL-10-producing B cells than those from a control group. Finally, dendritic plasmacytoid regulatory cells (pDCregs) are immune cells that carry the indoleamine 2,3-dioxygenase (IDO) enzyme, which reduces T effector cell activity and causes CD4+/CD25hi regulatory T cell polarization. IDO-mediated deprivation of tryptophan stops T cells from proliferating in the mid-G1 phase, resulting in immunological tolerance in combination with kynurenine's pro-apoptotic action. IDO plays a specific role in Th2 differentiation and is regulated positively in lymphocytes and dendritic cells after antigenic presentation and the functional complexing of CTLA-4/B7-1/B7-2. IDO also has a role in pathogen immunological responses, as it is upregulated by circulating nucleic acids (from both host and non-host genomes) via TLR4 and TLR9 activation, and it is involved in adaptive immunity processes that modify the inflammatory response. In the myenteric plexus of esophageal tissue from patients with achalasia, there was a higher frequency of pDCregs than in control tissues.

4.1.5 Autoantibodies

The increased incidence of circulating IgG antibodies against the myenteric plexus in most patients with achalasia has led to speculation that autoantibodies may play a role in the disease's development. Anti-myenteric autoantibody was also found to be absent in achalasia-free individuals, patients with Hirschsprung's disease, esophageal malignancy, peptic esophagitis, gastroesophageal reflux, or myasthenia gravis in studies. Nonetheless, Moses et al. concluded that these circulatory antibodies are more likely the outcome of a nonspecific reaction to the illness process than the cause of the sickness, which was corroborated by the discovery of comparable antibodies in individuals without achalasia. Autoantibodies against myenteric neurons were found in blood samples from individuals with achalasia, notably in carriers of the HLA DQA1*0103 and DQB1*0603 alleles, confirming the theories. Recent studies recently determined the levels of circulating anti-myenteric antibodies in serum from patients with achalasia. In the sera of idiopathic achalasia patients, the prevalence of nuclear or cytoplasmic circulating antibodies against the myenteric plexus was 63% and 100%, respectively, compared to 12% and 0% in the sera of healthy donors; additionally, most antibodies showed positive reaction in the nuclear and nucleolar compartments of cells in the myenteric plexus. Other autoantibodies, such as glutamic acid descarboxylase-65 (GAD65) antibody, have been found in serum from non-diabetic patients with achalasia, with a much higher frequency than in control participants (21% vs 2.5%). GAD65 is an enzyme found in GABAergic nerve terminals in the enteric nervous system that converts glutamic acid to gamma-aminobutyric acid. Antibodies to GAD65 are seen in about 80% of individuals with type 1 diabetes and 20% of patients with a variety of organ-specific neurological illnesses, such as myasthenia gravis, Lambert-Eaton syndrome, autoimmune dysautonomias, and encephalopathies. Approximately 40% of achalasia patients assessed in similar investigations had at least one other organ-specific autoantibody, such as thyroid or stomach parietal cell antibodies, and > 40% of patients had antinuclear antibodies (Table 4.4).

TABLE 4.4   Autoantibodies in Achalasia.

Generally against myenteric plexus
Often in HLA DQA1*0103—DQB1*0603 +
AntiGABAergic—Anti-GAD65 antibodies found
40% of achalasia patients have at least one other organ-specific antibody.

4.1.6 Genetics

Achalasia's growth and progression could be influenced by genetic factors. Achalasia may be inherited and so have a genetic component, as evidenced by the presence of familial cases. Achalasia has also been discovered to have statistical relationships with well-defined hereditary disorders. For example, a mutation in the ALADIN 12q13 gene, which is linked to Allgrove syndrome, causes clinical signs of achalasia, alacrima, and adrenocorticotrophic hormone-resistant adrenal insufficiency (Triple-A) in exons 1, 2, 7, 8, 10–14, and 16, as well as a poly(A) tract. Achalasia has also been linked to the MEN 2B syndrome, which is caused by a germline mutation in exon 16 (M918T) of the RET proto-oncogene on chromosome 10q11, which causes a methionine-threonine amino acid substitution in the tyrosine kinase domain, resulting in constitutive activation of the oncogene. The MEN 2 mutation can cause one of three types of cancer predisposition, all of which are inherited in an autosomal dominant manner: familial medullary thyroid carcinoma, MEN 2A, and MEN 2B. Achalasia has also been connected to Riley-Day syndrome (familial dysautonomia) and Smith-Lemli-Opitz syndrome syndrome (elevated amounts of 7- and 8-dehydrocholesterol due to reductase insufficiency). Achalasia with Hirschsprung's disease, commonly known as aganglionic megacolon, has also been described. Achalasia affects up to 2% of children with Down's syndrome, owing to a considerable reduction in the number of neurons in the esophageal plexus in this population. Finally, achalasia in children has been linked to congenital central hypoventilation syndrome. Due to the rarity of idiopathic achalasia, another method to genetic study of these cases has been to discover candidate genes by identifying single nucleotide polymorphisms (SNPs) and categorizing their clinical phenotype. The disease-related microsatellite (CA repeat) polymorphism has been discovered inside the 3'-untranslated region (UTR) of exon 29 of the neuronal nitric oxide synthase (NOS1) gene on human chromosome 12q24.2. Exome analysis of two siblings with infant-onset achalasia revealed homozygosity for a premature stop codon in the NOS1 gene (at residue Tyr1202, instead of at residue 1435). The shortened protein product has a poor folding ability, as well as NO generation and co-factor binding capacities, according to kinetic studies and molecular modeling. Endothelial NOS4a4a, inducible NOS22GA, and neuronal NOS29TT are some of the other NOS gene isoforms that have been revealed to have genetic polymorphisms. On chromosome 3p22, the gene for the receptor of vasoactive intestinal polypeptide (VIPR1) is found. VIPR1 is a member of the secretin receptor family, which includes immune cells (T cells, macrophages, and dendritic cells) as well as myenteric neurons in the distal esophagus and LES. It is highly polymorphic, and five SNPs, including (rs421558) intron-1, (rs437876) intron-4, (rs417387) intron-6, and (rs896 and rs9677) 3'-UTR, have been reported in patients with late achalasia. The IL-23 receptor (IL-23R) gene is found on chromosome 1p31, and the IL-23R protein encoded by it is expressed by Th17 cells and has been linked to chronic autoimmune diseases. An IL-23R gene polymorphism, in which arginine replaces glutamine at codon 381, was shown to be considerably more common in achalasia patients than in healthy controls in one investigation. The PTPN22 gene is found on chromosome 1p13.3-p13, within a region linked to autoimmune illness; the encoded protein, an intracellular lymphoid-specific tyrosine phosphatase (Lyp), is a downregulator of T cell activation. In girls of Spanish heritage, an SNP in the PTPN22 gene at position 1858C/T, which results in the replacement of arginine with tryptophan in codon 620, has been demonstrated to increase the incidence of achalasia [15,65]. Different autoimmune disorders, such as systemic lupus erythematosus, type 1 diabetes, ulcerative colitis, and asthma, have been linked to polymorphisms in the

IL10 gene; however, the GCC haplotype of the IL10 promoter has been linked to a decreased risk of achalasia. Finally, polymorphisms in the IL-33 gene, which encodes the IL-1 cytokine family member IL-33 and is known to play a critical role in chronic inflammatory autoimmune diseases, have been found to be more common in females with achalasia when compared to controls; the polymorphisms in question are the rs3939286 SNP and the rs7044343T/rs3939286A risk haplotype. Antigens of the human leukocyte antigen (HLA) class II have also been linked to autoimmune illnesses like SLE, Sjögren's syndrome, and other connective tissue diseases. Furthermore, T cell lymphocytes that identify particular class II antigens predominate in the myenteric infiltrates. HLA-DQ1 (HLA-DQB1*05:03 and HLA-DQB1*06:01), HLA-DQ1 (HLA-DQA1*01:03), and HLA-DQ1 (HLA-DQB1*03:01 and HLA-DQB1*03:04) have all been linked to achalasia. Many studies have found a link between this condition and numerous class II HLA antigens in Caucasians, including DQw1, DQA1*0103, DQB1*0601, DQB1*0602, DQB1*0603, DQB1*0601, DQB1*0502, and DQB1*0503 alleles. Furthermore, patients who carry the DQA1*0103 and DQB1*0603 alleles have a much greater incidence of anti-myenteric antibodies. An 8-residue insertion at position 227–234 in the cytoplasmic tail of HLA-DQ1 (encoded by HLA-DQB1*05:03 and HLA-DQB1*06:01) was identified as providing the highest risk for achalasia in a study of 1,068 instances of achalasia from Central Europe, Spain, and Italy. Two amino acid changes in the extracellular domain of HLA-DQ1 at position 41 (lysine encoded by HLA-DQA1*01:03) and position 45 (glutamic acid encoded by HLA-DQB1*03:01 and HLA-DQB1*03:04) have been identified as conferring achalasia risk separately. Furthermore, the HLA-DQ1 insertion has been identified as a major risk factor for achalasia, with a distinct north-south gradient among Europeans. The discovery that this insertion was less common in northern European populations than in southern European populations paralleled the disease's varied prevalence between populations. This geographic profile could be due to a genetic predisposition, putting some people at a higher chance of acquiring achalasia after being exposed to certain environmental conditions. It is worth noting that not all achalasia patients have the putative "predisposing" HLA, and not everyone with the HLA has the condition. As a result, the initial event that causes achalasia could be the result of a repeated assault caused by a neurotropic viral infection, most likely HSV-1, which causes a visible and chronic inflammation in the myenteric plexus at the perineural level. Because of a genetic susceptibility to develop a chronic auto-inflammatory response with the potential to advance to achalasia, not all infected patients will develop the condition.

TABLE 4.5   Mutations and Conditions Linked to Achalasia.

HLA-DQB1*05:03
HLA-DQB1*06:01
Mutation in 12q13 gene (Allgrove syndrome)
Mutation in exon 16, 10q11 of RET proto-oncogene (MEN 2B syndrome)
Riley-Day and Smith-Lemli-Opitz syndromes
VIPR1 polymorphisms
IL-23R, IL-33 polymorphisms
Hirschsprung's disease
Down's syndrome (2% prevalence)
Congenital central hypoventilation syndrome

4.2 PATHOPHYSIOLOGY OF ACHALASIA: A PROPOSED MODEL

This proposed model of achalasia pathophysiology was modified from Furuzawa-Carballeda (Table 4.6): It develops from an initial active or latent infectious insult, most likely involving a neurotropic virus, such as the herpes family of viruses or varicella zoster, which have a preference for squamous epithelium and neurons and may cause ganglion cell damage limited to the esophagus.

TABLE 4.6 A Step-by-Step Proposed Model of Pathophysiology in Achalasia.

1. Initial active/latent insult by neurotropic viruses, causing limited damage
2. Aggressive inflammatory response in genetically susceptible patients
3. Damage mediated by TGF, IL-4, IL-13, and pro-fibrogenic cytokines
4. In case of chronic infection and genetic tendency to autoimmunity, disease progresses
5. Immune-mediated inhibitory neuronal loss and fiber degeneration
6. Anti-myenteric autoantibodies in serum support an autoimmune etiology
7. Loss of inhibitory ganglion in the myenteric plexus caused by autoinflammation, nerve degeneration, plexitis, ganglionitis, microvascular abnormalities

4.3 FURTHER READING

Akiho, H., E. Ihara, Y. Motomura, and K. Nakamura, "Cytokine-induced alterations of gastrointestinal motility in gastrointestinal disorders," *World Journal of Gastrointestinal Pathophysiology*, vol. 2, no. 5, pp. 72–81, 2011.

Boeckxstaens, G. E., "Novel mechanism for impaired nitrergic relaxation in achalasia," *Gut*, vol. 55, no. 3, pp. 304–5, 2006.

Boeckxstaens, G. E., "Achalasia: virus-induced euthanasia of neurons?" *The American Journal of Gastroenterology*, vol. 103, no. 7, pp. 1610–12, 2008.

Boeckxstaens, G. E., G. Zaninotto, and J. E. Richter, "Achalasia," *The Lancet*, vol. 383, no. 9911, pp. 83–93, 2014.

Bruley des Varannes, S., J. Chevalier, S. Pimont, et al., "Serum from achalasia patients alters neurochemical coding in the myenteric plexus and nitric oxide mediated motor response in normal human fundus," *Gut*, vol. 55, no. 3, pp. 319–26, 2006.

Clark, S. B., T. W. Rice, R. R. Tubbs, J. E. Richter, and J. R. Goldblum, "The nature of the myenteric infiltrate in achalasia: an immunohistochemical analysis," *The American Journal of Surgical Pathology*, vol. 24, no. 8, pp. 1153–8, 2000.

Dhamija, R., K. M. Tan, S. J. Pittock, A. Foxx-Orenstein, E. Benarroch, and V. A. Lennon, "Serologic profiles aiding the diagnosis of autoimmune gastrointestinal dysmotility," *Clinical Gastroenterology and Hepatology*, vol. 6, no. 9, pp. 988–92, 2008.

Facco, M., P. Brun, I. Baesso, et al., "T cells in the myenteric plexus of achalasia patients show a skewed TCR repertoire and react to HSV-1 antigens," *American Journal of Gastroenterology*, vol. 103, no. 7, pp. 1598–609, 2008.

Furuzawa-Carballeda, J., G. Fonseca-Camarillo, G. Lima, and J. K. Yamamoto-Furusho, "Indoleamine 2,3-dioxygenase: expressing cells in inflammatory bowel disease—a cross-sectional study," *Clinical and Developmental Immunology*, vol. 2013, Article ID 278035, 14 pages, 2013.

Furuzawa-Carballeda, J., G. Lima, J. Jakez-Ocampo, and L. Llorente, "Indoleamine 2,3-dioxygenase-expressing peripheral cells in rheumatoid arthritis and systemic lupus erythematosus: a cross-sectional study," *European Journal of Clinical Investigation*, vol. 41, no. 10, pp. 1037–46, 2011.

Furuzawa-Carballeda, J., J. Sánchez-Guerrero, J. L. Betanzos, et al., "Differential cytokine expression and regulatory cells in patients with primary and secondary Sjögren's syndrome," *Scandinavian Journal of Immunology*, vol. 80, no. 6, pp. 432–40, 2014.

Ganem, D., A. Kistler, and J. DeRisi, "Achalasia and viral infection: new insights from veterinary medicine," *Science Translational Medicine*, vol. 2, no. 33, Article ID 33ps24, 2010.

Ghoshal, U. C., S. B. Daschakraborty, and R. Singh, "Pathogenesis of achalasia cardia," *World Journal of Gastroenterology*, vol. 18, no. 24, pp. 3050–7, 2012.

Kallel-Sellami, M., S. Karoui, H. Romdhane, et al., "Circulating antimyenteric autoantibodies in Tunisian patients with idiopathic achalasia," *Diseases of the Esophagus*, vol. 26, no. 8, pp. 782–7, 2013.

Kilic, A., A. M. Krasinskas, S. R. Owens, J. D. Luketich, R. J. Landreneau, and M. J. Schuchert, "Variations in inflammation and nerve fiber loss reflect different subsets of achalasia patients," *Journal of Surgical Research*, vol. 143, no. 1, pp. 177–82, 2007.

Korn, T., E. Bettelli, M. Oukka, and V. K. Kuchroo, "IL-17 and Th17 cells," *Annual Review of Immunology*, vol. 27, pp. 485–517, 2009.

Kraichely, R. E., G. Farrugia, S. J. Pittock, D. O. Castell, and V. A. Lennon, "Neural autoantibody profile of primary achalasia," *Digestive Diseases and Sciences*, vol. 55, no. 2, pp. 307–11, 2010.

Latiano, A., R. de Giorgio, U. Volta et al., "HLA and enteric antineuronal antibodies in patients with achalasia," *Neurogastroenterology & Motility*, vol. 18, no. 7, pp. 520–5, 2006.

Mayberry, J. F., "Epidemiology and demographics of achalasia," *Gastrointestinal Endoscopy Clinics of North America*, vol. 11, no. 2, pp. 235–47, 2001.

Niwamoto, H., E. Okamoto, J. Fujimoto, M. Takeuchi, J.-I. Furuyama, and Y. Yamamoto, "Are human herpes viruses or measles virus associated with esophageal achalasia?" *Digestive Diseases and Sciences*, vol. 40, no. 4, pp. 859–64, 1995.

Pandolfino, J. E., M. A. Kwiatek, T. Nealis, W. Bulsiewicz, J. Post, and P. J. Kahrilas, "Achalasia: a new clinically relevant classification by high-resolution manometry," *Gastroenterology*, vol. 135, no. 5, pp. 1526–33, 2008.

Petersen, R. P., A. V. Martin, C. A. Pellegrini, and B. K. Oelschlager, "Synopsis of investigations into proposed theories on the etiology of achalasia," *Diseases of the Esophagus*, vol. 25, no. 4, pp. 305–10, 2012.

Raymond, L., B. Lach, and F. M. Shamji, "Inflammatory aetiology of primary oesophageal achalasia: an immunohistochemical and ultrastructural study of Auerbach's plexus," *Histopathology*, vol. 35, no. 5, pp. 445–53, 1999.

Ruiz-de-León, A., J. Mendoza, C. Sevilla-Mantilla, et al., "Myenteric antiplexus antibodies and class II HLA in achalasia," *Digestive Diseases and Sciences*, vol. 47, no. 1, pp. 15–19, 2002.

Simera, I., D. Moher, J. Hoey, K. F. Schulz, and D. G. Altman, "A catalogue of reporting guidelines for health research," *European Journal of Clinical Investigation*, vol. 40, no. 1, pp. 35–53, 2010.

Sinagra, E., E. Gallo, F. Mocciaro et al., "JC virus, helicobacter pylori, and oesophageal achalasia: preliminary results from a retrospective case-control study," *Digestive Diseases and Sciences*, vol. 58, no. 5, pp. 1433–4, 2013.

Willis, T., *Pharmaceutice Rationalis Sive Diatribe de Medicamentorum Operationibus in Humano Corpore*, Hagae Comitis, London, UK, 1674.

Wong, R. K. H., C. L. Maydonovitch, S. J. Metz, and J. R. Baker Jr., "Significant DQw1 association in achalasia," *Digestive Diseases and Sciences*, vol. 34, no. 3, pp. 349–52, 1989.

Clinical Overview of Achalasia

Giuseppe Fuggi, Francesca Russo, and Rocco Granata

Contents

5.1 INTRODUCTION

One of the staples of our way of approaching clinical problems is using a multidisciplinary team (MDT), an integrated effort of specialist physicians, each putting forward his or her own knowledge for the betterment of patients. In achalasia, an uncoordinated clinical approach is definitely not productive and often inconclusive, with many patients getting diagnosed late. An Upper GI team dedicated to the diagnoses of motility disorders should primarily be made up of clinicians, mainly gastroenterologists who put forward the first clinical suspicion and, in the end, make a definite diagnosis by performing high-resolution manometry (HRM), a relatively new technique deemed, at the time of writing, the new diagnostic gold standard; in the MDT, though, a main supporting role is that of endoscopists and radiologists, the latter mainly using computed tomography (CT) and ultrasound, who basically rule out potential other causes with similar clinical appearances, such as malignancies, acid reflux with peptic strictures or structural disorders like esophageal rings and webs, eosinophilic esophagitis, etc. Last but not least, specialist surgeons are of course an integral, important part of the dedicated MDT, often the ending point of the patient's journey. As we will see in the next section, a nutritionist should be on the team as well, to correct the many nutritional imbalances

DOI: 10.1201/9781003320302-5

that are so often found and even more often guiltily overlooked in patients with severe dysphagia or eating impairment. Even though a combined clinical and manometrical approach may theoretically allow a correct diagnosis, definite diagnosis being made by HRM as said before, there are nowadays so many tools a clinician may use not only to make a differential diagnosis, but to assess and even grade a specific disease, that it would be foolish not to use them. The role of diagnostic endoscopy, namely, esophagogastroduodenoscopy (EGD) is well established in the diagnostic algorithm of achalasia, but EGD is essentially used to rule out pseudoachalasia, due to malignant neoplasms or other structural problems such as those cited before, considering that up to 40% of patients undergoing EGD will end up having a normal endoscopy. Imaging, on the other hand, while serving as an excellent tool to rule out other potential diagnosis, especially using CT or contrast-enhanced CT (CECT), has always found its supporting role in the diagnosis of achalasia in the old-but-gold barium esophagogram, which is the main theme of this book. As said in the introduction, though, our aim is to revamp this often unjustly neglected technique, highlighting its innumerable advantages, using all the latest advancements in radiographic technology, which allow a real-time morphodynamical analysis. As extensively explained in the next chapters, our efforts are toward establishing a clinically oriented, radiographic grading system that is compatible with the clinical-manometrical Chicago Classification and would be of huge support to the clinical, endoscopic, and manometrical approaches.

5.2 CLINICAL FINDINGS

Achalasia may at first present with a number of different symptoms that, combined together, massively deteriorate the patient's quality of life, work productivity, and functional status (Table 5.1). A classical clinical presentation of achalasia is as progressive dysphagia to both solids and liquids, with patients reporting symptoms in 82–100% of cases. Another very common symptom (76–91%) is regurgitation. Heartburn, the hallmark of the total antithesis of achalasia, gastroesophageal reflux disease (GERD), can be explained by retention of acidic or noxious food contents or by endoluminal bacterial fermentation and lactate production. The presence of heartburn in 27% to 42% of patients with achalasia often leads patients to be misdiagnosed with GERD and consequently treated with proton pump inhibitor (PPI); incorrect diagnoses of GERD often lead to a late or very late diagnosis of achalasia, which is generally made when symptoms are very evident and unmistakable. Chest pain is present, too, in 25–64% of patients. Now, while regurgitation and dysphagia, the commonest symptoms, tend to be present in patients of all ages, heartburn and chest pain are much more frequent in younger patients. Even though slightly rarer, hiccup may be present, due to esophageal dilation and stimulation of vagal afferent fibers. Patients with a body mass index [BMI] ≥30 are more likely to develop choking or vomiting symptoms, while patients with type III achalasia and women present more frequently with chest pain. Many studies show that a share of patients between 35% and 91% reports weight loss during initial presentation, with an average weight loss of 9.0 ± 7.2 kgs. Often, after pneumatic dilation, patients tend to regain the lost weight, with just a mere 6% reporting a continuing weight loss. Of course, a considerable weight loss brings huge nutritional implications with itself, something that is often overlooked due to the lack of multidisciplinary work or, even worse, for "cultural" reasons. Another distinctive feature of patients with achalasia is their diagnostic latency: the duration of the symptoms, before the diagnostic process, ranges between two and 20 years; this is pretty much confirmed by our own clinical practice, the longest wait between symptom onset and diagnosis being 18 years, in a 48-year-old woman. Achalasia may have extraesophageal manifestations, too, the most common being pulmonary complications. More than half of the patients suffer with functional or structural pulmonary abnormalities that are mainly due to recurrent aspiration or tracheal compression from a dilated esophagus; a so-called bull frog neck appearance may develop in cases of extreme dilation and distortion of the cervical esophagus, this leading to tracheal obstruction above the larynx and associated stridor. Delayed gastric emptying and gallbladder dysfunction are often reported by patients with achalasia, which might be due to a distant effect of the selective defect of vagal ganglionic neurons, which might affect other organs or portions of the gastrointestinal tract; this, though, remains very much a hypothesis still to this day. This wide spectrum of symptoms of achalasia reported here is something to know and keep in mind all the time, because the aforementioned diagnostic latency, long waits for years after the onset of symptoms, might be due to misinterpretation of typical findings, something that happens more often than not, rather than atypical presentations.

TABLE 5.1 Prevalence of Symptoms in Achalasia.

PRESENTING SYMPTOM	PATIENTS REPORTING THE SYMPTOM
Dysphagia	82–100%
Regurgitation	76–91%
Weight loss	35–91%
Chest pain	25–64%
Heartburn	27–42%
Nocturnal cough	37%
Aspiration	8%

5.3 DIAGNOSTIC ENDOSCOPY

The first natural step, for a patient referred with dysphagia, is to conduct an esophagogastroduodenoscopy, essentially to exclude the presence of structural abnormalities such as esophageal carcinoma, peptic strictures with acid reflux, rings, webs, or eosinophilic esophagitis. However, even though an endoscopic diagnosis of achalasia is made in just about a third of all patients with achalasia, its sensitivity increases dramatically with the progression of the disease. The main role of diagnostic endoscopy is to rule out other possible causes for the symptoms, giving the operator the possibility to biopsy. Typical sign is the increased resistance at the gastroesophageal junction, that is however still relatively easy to pass with the endoscope (Figure 5.1). Esophageal dilation and food/secretion retention are found in the advanced stages of the disease. The esophageal mucosa usually appears normal, although sometimes inflammation or ulceration caused by retained food can be demonstrated (Figure 5.2).

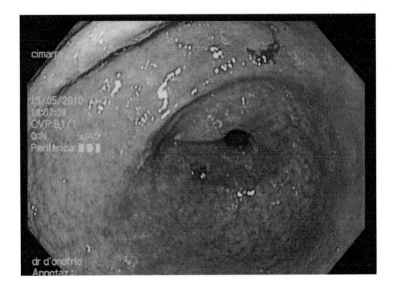

FIGURE 5.1 Endoscopic image showing the narrowing of the lumen at the LES.

Source: Image courtesy of Biondo Francesco Giuseppe, MD.

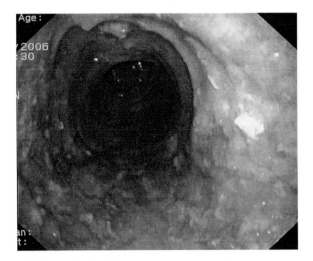

FIGURE 5.2 Endoscopic image showing residual food, inflammation, and ulcerations in the esophageal lumen.

Source: Image courtesy of Biondo Francesco Giuseppe, MD.

5.4 HIGH-RESOLUTION MANOMETRY AND CHICAGO CLASSIFICATION

Generally, when endoscopy is reported as normal, esophageal manometry is the immediate next step for the detection of esophageal motility disorders. Very important improvements have been put in place the last few years, in the manometric sensor technology, manometric data display, and manometric data analysis. In comparison with conventional manometry, high-resolution manometry (HRM) provides improved and more detailed information on esophageal motility and is, as of today, considered the gold standard in the diagnosis of esophageal motility disorders and, of course, achalasia. This technique, compared with conventional manometry, uses more sensors (20–36), dramatically decreasing the spacing between them (1 cm versus 3–6 cm). The pressure signals are converted in color plots that create what is referred to as pressure topography, which enables a quick and intuitional interpretation. The Chicago Classification is a scheme specifically developed to allow an objective analysis of HRM metrics and topography. This is a hierarchical system of analysis, comprehensively divided into four major categories, each based on specific patterns of LES relaxation and esophageal body motility, the first of them being of interest to us: incomplete LES relaxation, namely, achalasia or esophagogastric junction outflow obstruction. HRM and, consequently, the Chicago Classification are so widespread, so commonly used in clinical practice and studies that they provided innumerable and significant insights in regard to esophageal motility disorders and achalasia. This is one of the main reasons that we, as a research group, felt compelled to help dynamical radiography move forward in the same direction, giving it a new dimension it never had before. Technically speaking, using the Chicago Classification, achalasia is diagnosed when an elevated median integrated relaxation pressure (IRP), in combination with failed peristalsis or spasm, is found. Practically, HRM led to the recognition of three different achalasia patterns or subtypes, with different manometric and clinical features and, more importantly, different prognostic outcomes (Figure 5.3): subtype I, hypotonic or classic, with no pressure waves are recorded in the distal esophagus; subtype II, characterized by panesophageal pressurizations, with patients most likely to report weight loss; subtype III, spastic, in which at least 20% of swallows reveal rapidly propagating or spastic simultaneous contractions; patients here are more likely to report chest pain, rather than weight loss. The most important consideration to make about this relatively new classification is that the treatment outcome depends on the diagnosed subtype that can be used to predict treatment response. The vast majority of the studies observe that the best treatment response is reported in patients with type II achalasia (95–96%), while the worst response in patients with type III achalasia (29–70%). A suggestion as to why these three subtypes behave and respond differently can be partially found in many studies regarding the pathological aspect of the disease: subtype I and II both show increased aganglionosis and neuronal loss at the myenteric plexus, while subtype III shows preserved ganglion cells (Table 5.2). Different grades of myenteric inflammation and fibrosis are, however, found in all three subtypes, but they vary greatly from patient to patient.

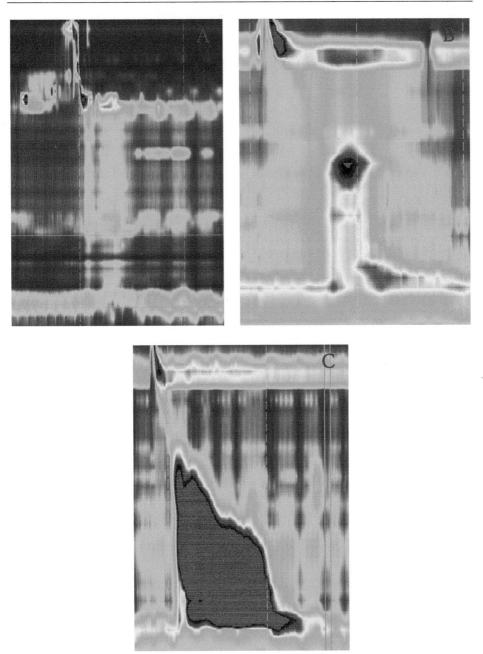

FIGURE 5.3 High-Resolution manometry patterns: (a) Hypotonic, (b) Panpressurizing, (c) Spastic.

Source: Image courtesy of Rocco Granata, MD.

TABLE 5.2 Manometric, Clinical, and Histologic Differences among the Three Achalasia Subtypes.

ACHALASIA SUBTYPE	MANOMETRIC FINDINGS	CLINICAL FINDINGS	HISTOLOGIC FINDINGS
I	Elevated median IRP (>15 mmHg) 100% failed peristalsis (DCI<100 mmHg/s/cm)		Increased aganglionosis and neuronal loss
II	Elevated median IRP (>15 mmHg) Panesophageal panpressurization >20% of swallows	Most likely to report weight loss	Increased aganglionosis and neuronal loss
III	Elevated median IRP (>15 mmHg) Premature contractions >20% swallows with DCI > 450 mmHg/s/cm	Least likely to report weight loss More likely to report chest pain	Preserved ganglion cells

DCI = distal contractile integral; IRP = integrated relaxation pressure

5.5 TREATMENT

It is not the scope of this book to treat the surgical approach to achalasia into detail, but, as we are trying to establish a new, clinically oriented way of interpreting radiographic images, we think it is mandatory for the imaging specialist to know how the three different achalasia subtypes are treated, their different prognosis, ending up considering achalasia as three slightly different syndromes and not just one disease. The first and most important statement to make about the treatment of achalasia is that, currently, there is no drug and endoscopic or surgical procedure capable of halting or reversing the immunologically driven plexopathy, the main cause of progressing idiopathic achalasia. What treatments can do, however, is to try and alleviate the esophageal outflow obstruction, reducing stress on the esophagogastric junction, slowing or potentially halting the progressive dilation of the esophageal lumen, which is mainly responsible for the long-term morbidity of the disease and a common trait between the three achalasia subtypes. What does actually vary, even dramatically, between the three subtypes is the associated pattern of contractility, going from totally absent in subtype I to spastic in subtype III; consequently, a treating approach should be tailored on the phenotype of the patient, especially considering statements found in literature that link even treatment success to specific phenotypes: treatment outcomes are found to be best in type II achalasia, with excellent treatment outcomes ranging from 90 to 100% and likely worst in type III achalasia. Each clinical subtype, or phenotype, has to be considered singularly, each with

TABLE 5.3   Preferred Treatment Options for Each Achalasia Subtype.

ACHALASIA SUBTYPE	PREFERRED TREATMENTS	COMMENTS, RATIONALE
I	PD, LHM, POEM	- All are efficacious. - Expect more reflux after POEM, especially with hiatal hernia. - Extending myotomy proximal to the LES is probably unnecessary and can lead to diverticula at the myotomy site.
II	PD	- PD, LHM, POEM are all highly efficacious; PD has the least morbidity and cost. - Anticipate repeat dilations over the years. - Extending myotomy proximal to the LES is probably unnecessary and can lead to diverticula at the myotomy site.
III	POEM	Calibrate the length of myotomy to the spastic segment as imaged on HRM.

its preferred treatment, rationale, and unique optimal management strategy, as shown in Table 5.3.

Now, considering drug treatments to reduce LES pressure, there are very little supporting data and the few studies found in literature often date before the introduction of achalasia subtyping, therefore making many considerations and suppositions impossible. The most studied drugs are, however, nitrates, calcium channel blockers, botulinum toxin, and, a recent introduction, 5'-phosphodiesterase inhibitors. Smooth muscle relaxants may be used as a symptomatic relief treatment but cannot be considered durable therapies, because they often cause side effects, some of them intolerable, and they, after all, are not capable of halting the progression of esophageal dilation and food retention. Using botulinum toxin injection into the LES, 66% of patients show marked clinical benefit; many, though, relapse within the first year and it is proved that repeated treatments diminish botulinum toxin effectiveness, in some cases making potential surgical interventions much more difficult than in the first place. Often, these treatments are used in patients with severe comorbidity and not really fit for other therapeutic strategies. Until recent times, the only considerable and durable therapeutic choices were pneumatic dilation (PD) and laparoscopic Heller myotomy (LHM). Pneumatic dilation is performed by using a 30-, 35-, or 40-mm cylindrical balloon fluoroscopically positioned at the LES, then manually inflated using a manometer (Figure 5.4). The surgical alternative to PD used as a standard is LHM, a technique in which a surgical division of circular muscle layer of the LES is performed. Many surgeons recommend that the myotomy be anterior and about 70 mm in overall length, extending at least 20 mm onto the gastric cardia and 50 mm onto the tubular esophagus. As this often tends to create gastroesophageal reflux, a partial fundoplication is generally added to LHM. Many studies, although dating before the introduction of the

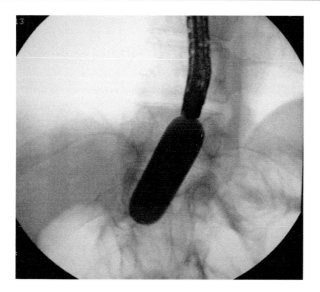

FIGURE 5.4   Intraoperatory fluoroscopy frame of endoscopic pneumatic dilation.

Source: Image courtesy of Biondo Francesco Giuseppe, MD.

Chicago Classification, have compared LHM with PD, concluding that both were about 90% effective without a significant difference between them; retrospective analysis, after the introduction of achalasia subtyping have of course been made and the efficacy of PD for treating type II achalasia has found to be 100%. Now, considering the costs of PD are dramatically lower than those of LIIM and that the risk of perforation between techniques is comparable, about 1% in expert hands, this makes PD the preferred initial treatment for type II achalasia. The introduction and subsequent widespread adoption of the per-oral endoscopic myotomy (POEM) procedure has been hailed as a major innovation in the treatment approach to achalasia. The POEM procedure is substantially performed by making a mucosal incision in the mid-esophagus and creating a submucosal tunnel to the gastric cardia using a standard endoscope and electrocautery. From within the submucosal tunnel, a circular muscle layer myotomy is performed, starting at the gastric cardia and progressing proximally across the LES. This is what makes POEM unique and especially useful for patients with subtype III achalasia: the myotomy can be extended longer if needed, potentially involving the entire length of smooth muscle esophagus. Subtype III achalasia can benefit greatly from this, considering that treatments limited to the LES have worse outcomes. Recent studies who support this hypothesis reported a weighted pooled response rate of 92% in type III achalasia with the length of myotomy averaging 17.2 cm. Of course, this wide range of treatment options is rarely available to any patient, anytime and anywhere. The same can be said of the clinical expertise and diagnostic tools described before; that is why Upper GI MDTs are needed, to allow the diagnosis and the best available treatment, or referral, of patients (Table 5.4).

TABLE 5.4   Diagnostic and Therapeutic Pathways in Achalasia.

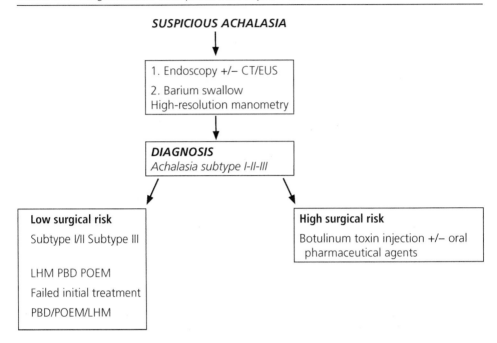

5.6 FURTHER READING

Annese V, Caruso N, Accadia L, Gabbrielli A, Modoni S, Frusciante V, Federici T. Gallbladder function and gastric liquid emptying in achalasia. *Dig Dis Sci.* 1991;36:1116–20.

Boeckxstaens GE, Annese V, des Varannes SB, Chaussade S, Costantini M, et al. Pneumatic dilation versus laparoscopic Heller's myotomy for idiopathic achalasia. *N Engl J Med.* 2011;364:1807–16.

Camacho-Lobato L, Katz PO, Eveland J, Vela M, Castell DO. Vigorous achalasia: original description requires minor change. *J Clin Gastroenterol.* 2001;33:375–7.

Csendes A, Smok G, Braghetto I, González P, Henríquez A, Csendes P, Pizurno D. Histological studies of Auerbach's plexuses of the oesophagus, stomach, jejunum, and colon in patients with achalasia of the oesophagus: correlation with gastric acid secretion, presence of parietal cells and gastric emptying of solids. *Gut.* 1992;33:150–4.

De Giorgio R, Guerrini S, Barbara G, Stanghellini V, De Ponti F, Corinaldesi R, Moses PL, Sharkey KA, Mawe GM. Inflammatory neuropathies of the enteric nervous system. *Gastroenterology.* 2004;126:1872–83.

Eckardt VF. Clinical presentations and complications of achalasia. *Gastrointest Endosc Clin N Am.* 2001;11:281–92, vi.

Eckardt VF, Köhne U, Junginger T, Westermeier T. Risk factors for diagnostic delay in achalasia. *Dig Dis Sci.* 1997;42:580–5.

Eckardt VF, Krause J, Bolle D. Gastrointestinal transit and gastric acid secretion in patients with achalasia. *Dig Dis Sci.* 1989;34:665–71.

Eckardt VF, Schmitt T, Kanzler G. Transabdominal ultrasonography in achalasia. *Scand J Gastroenterol*. 2004;39:634–7.

Eckardt VF, Stauf B, Bernhard G. Chest pain in achalasia: patient characteristics and clinical course. *Gastroenterology*. 1999;116:1300–4.

Fisichella PM, Raz D, Palazzo F, Niponmick I, Patti MG. Clinical, radiological, and manometric profile in 145 patients with untreated achalasia. *World J Surg*. 2008;32:1974–9.

Fontanella G et al. A proposal for a new prognostic grading system in achalasia using dynamic barium swallow: the FBF score. *EMJ Radiol*. 2021;2(1):34–6.

Gockel I, Eckardt VF, Schmitt T, Junginger T. Pseudoachalasia: a case series and analysis of the literature. *Scand J Gastroenterol*. 2005;40:378–85.

Goldenberg SP, Burrell M, Fette GG, Vos C, Traube M. Classic and vigorous achalasia: a comparison of manometric, radiographic, and clinical findings. *Gastroenterology*. 1991;101:743–8.

Hirano I, Tatum RP, Shi G, Sang Q, Joehl RJ, Kahrilas PJ. Manometric heterogeneity in patients with idiopathic achalasia. *Gastroenterology*. 2001;120:789–98.

Khan AK, Kumbhari V, Ngamruengphong S, Ismail M, Chen YI, et al. Is POEM the answer for management of spastic esophageal disorders? A systematic review and meta-analysis. *Dig Dis Sci*. 2017;62:35–4.

Liu W, Fackler W, Rice TW, Richter JE, Achkar E, Goldblum JR. The pathogenesis of pseudoachalasia: a clinicopathologic study of 13 cases of a rare entity. *Am J Surg Pathol*. 2002;26:784–8.

Lynch KL, Pandolfino JE, Howden CW, Kahrilas PJ. Major complications of pneumatic dilation and Heller myotomy for achalasia: single center experience and systematic review of the literature. *Am J Gastroenterol*. 2012;107:1817–25.

Makharia GK, Seith A, Sharma SK, Sinha A, Goswami P, Aggarwal A, Puri K, Sreenivas V. Structural and functional abnormalities in lungs in patients with achalasia. *Neurogastroenterol Motil*. 2009;42:603–8, e20.

Massey BT, Hogan WJ, Dodds WJ, Dantas RO. Alteration of the upper esophageal sphincter belch reflex in patients with achalasia. *Gastroenterology*. 1992;103:1574–9.

Mikaeli J, Farrokhi F, Bishehsari F, Mahdavinia M, Malekzadeh R. Gender effect on clinical features of achalasia: a prospective study. *BMC Gastroenterol*. 2006;6:12.

Moonen A, Annese V, Belmans A, Bredenoord AJ, Bruley des Varannes S, et al. Long-term results of the European achalasia trial: a multicenter randomised controlled trial comparing pneumatic dilation versus laparoscopic Heller myotomy. *Gut*. 2016;65:732–9.

Pandolfino JE, Gawron AJ. Achalasia a systematic review. *JAMA*. 2015;313(18):1841–52. Very current systematic review of the epidemiology, pathogenesis, and management of achalasia.

Pandolfino JE, Kwiatek MA, Nealis T, Bulsiewicz W, Post J, Kahrilas PJ. Achalasia: a new clinically relevant classification by high-resolution manometry. *Gastroenterology*. 2008;135:1526–33.

Patel DA, Lappas BM, Vaezi MF. An overview of achalasia and its subtypes. *Gastroenterol Hepatol (N Y)*. 2017;13(7):411–21.

Seeman H, Traube M. Hiccups and achalasia. *Ann Intern Med*. 1991;115:711–12.

Smart HL, Foster PN, Evans DF, Slevin B, Atkinson M. Twenty four hour oesophageal acidity in achalasia before and after pneumatic dilatation. *Gut*. 1987;28:883–7.

Spechler SJ, Souza RF, Rosenberg SJ, Ruben RA, Goyal RK. Heartburn in patients with achalasia. *Gut*. 1995;37:305–8.

Vaezi MF, Baker ME, Achkar E, Richter JE. Timed barium oesophagram: better predictor of long term success after pneumatic dilation in achalasia than symptom assessment. *Gut*. 2002;50:765–70.

Wright RA, Swan P. Gastric emptying in achalasia. *Scand J Gastroenterol*. 1991;26:798–800.

Fluoroscopy and Dynamic Barium Swallow

6

Simona Borrelli

Contents

6.1 INTRODUCTION

In this chapter, we are finally entering into the core of this book, morphodynamic imaging of the esophagus applied to achalasia. The techniques, or rather protocols, we are going to describe in the next few pages have all been developed by our group through extensive practice, with daily and tailored modifications, then used in clinical practice. Although many of the things we will discuss will be mainly based on dynamical or, as we prefer to define it, morphodynamic imaging, we do understand that direct digital devices with cine modality are still not the norm and not equally available anywhere; that is why we will present a static acquisition protocol as well. Timed barium esophagogram will be treated, too, a static, quick, and easy-to-perform technique that is very useful for post-therapeutic assessment. Even though our approach to the matter of barium swallow is rather one of moving forward, aimed at producing images that are more useful than just 'beautiful' to watch, we do not underestimate the value of the classic barium esophagogram and its use in routine studies. Our morphodynamic protocol should not be mistaken for something to be used routinely in all patients, but rather it should be performed only in patients

DOI: 10.1201/9781003320302-6

with certified motility disorders, considering the higher radiation dose and exposure times dynamical imaging determines. We strongly advise, though, using morphodynamic imaging whenever possible in patients with certain motility disorders, not exclusively achalasia. The analysis of the upper GI should ideally be complete, from pharynx to duodenum, but generally and especially in patients with achalasia or motility disorders, we include the stomach only when evident anomalies are present, focusing our evaluation on swallowing, esophageal emptying, esophageal morphology and motility, evaluation of the gastroesophageal (GE) junction, and assessment for gastroesophageal reflux (GER). Patients who have undergone recent esophageal or gastric surgery or recent trauma, or who are unable to cooperate with the examination are, however, not candidates for this kind of evaluation. Relevant patient history should be obtained prior to the procedure to determine the appropriate type of procedure and contrast medium. In these instances, assuming that the patient can cooperate, a single-contrast examination should be performed.

6.2 CONTRAST MEDIA AND TECHNIQUE

Rumple described the use of liquid contrast media (bismuth subnitrate) for opacifying the esophagus in 1897. However, this subnitrate form of bismuth was shown to be poisonous when reduced to a subnitrite form, necessitating a quest for safer contrast agents. Walter B. Cannon, a pioneering radiologist, was the first to report the use of barium sulfate for GI fluoroscopy in 1904, and by 1910, barium was being promoted as the standard contrast medium for GI examinations. The natural mineral barite contains barium sulfate, which is a white, crystalline, odorless solid. Barium's atomic number of 56 makes it suitable for absorbing X-rays. Barium has a strong chemical reactivity and is harmful to humans in water-soluble forms. Fortunately, due to its extremely low water solubility, barium sulfate may be employed safely as an intraluminal GI contrast agent. It should be noted that barium's 'liquid' state is not a solution, but rather a suspension of barium particles temporarily floating in water. To re-suspend the barium particles, a pre-prepared barium product must be forcefully shaken in its container before use, as experienced GI fluoroscopists are well aware (Figure 6.1). Sedimentation is the phenomenon of barium settling from its suspension, which can be minimized by utilizing tiny barium particles. Simultaneously, tiny particle size enhances barium viscosity. Over the last century, barium suspensions used to demonstrate the GI tract have seen tremendous improvements. Unadulterated barium sulfate clots or rather, flocculates, hindering an accurate evaluation of the intestine. Although chemical specifications for commercial barium suspensions are available, the precise compositions of proprietary barium solutions are not. Anti-clumping, anti-foaming, suspending, preservative, and flavoring compounds are applied to barium sulfate particles. The creation of barium preparations with varied viscosities has tremendously aided swallowing assessments. Because barium suspensions are non-Newtonian fluids, their viscosity changes with flow rate. As a result, barium viscosity is a thickness and flowing metric that cannot be calculated with a spin viscometer. For long of the twentieth century, the barium swallow was a single-contrast examination in which the patient ingested low-density barium to distend the pharyngeal and esophageal lumens with a single stream

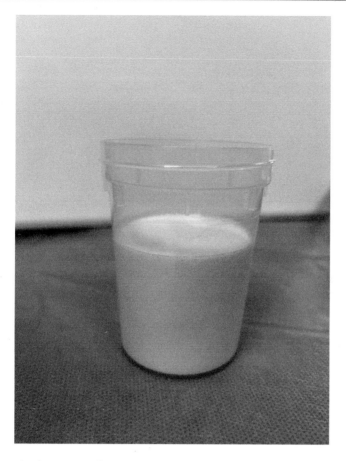

FIGURE 6.1   A barium suspension. Vigorous shaking right before examination is mandatory to avoid flocculation.

of thin barium. The single-contrast approach allowed for the identification of pharyngeal and esophageal strictures, contour abnormalities (such as ulcers or tumors), and big protruded lesions visible en face as radiolucent flaws in the barium column. This approach, however, did not allow for the observation of tiny protruded or depressed mucosal lesions, and so had a limited sensitivity for identifying inflammatory or neoplastic diseases. The idea of combining air and barium to see the mucosal surface of the GI tract was initially proposed in the early twentieth century. For excellent mucosa coating on double-contrast GI examinations, high-density, low-viscosity barium products were developed, notably for the study of the stomach and colon. These double-contrast examinations, however, were later found to significantly increase the identification of mild mucosal abnormalities in the pharynx and esophagus. Igor Laufer of the University of Pennsylvania was a key proponent of the double-contrast method for increasing the identification of mucosal lesions in the esophagus in the 1970s. He presented a simplified technique for performing double-contrast esophagrams in his classic text, *Double Contrast Gastrointestinal Radiology with*

Endoscopic Correlation, first published in 1977, in which the patient ingested an effervescent agent that released carbon dioxide gas into the gastric lumen and then continuously swallowed a high-density barium suspension to coat the mucosa for double-contrast views of the esophagus. This approach dramatically enhanced the identification of reflux esophagitis, infectious esophagitis, various esophagitides, and esophageal cancer, as well as the distinction between benign and malignant strictures (see later sections). Despite the benefits of the double-contrast technique for visualizing the mucosa, it was discovered that swallowing a low-density barium suspension continuously in the prone, right anterior oblique (RAO) position produced better esophageal distention for visualization of rings and strictures, particularly in the distal esophagus. Ott et al. produced a series of studies between 1982 and 1986 demonstrating that prone, single-contrast views significantly enhanced the identification of distal esophageal rings and strictures, even those missed on upright double-contrast views or even endoscopy. As a result, the barium study is now conducted in two phases, with upright double-contrast and prone single-contrast images of the esophagus. Although high-density barium is better for demonstrating anatomic structures, swallowing function is tested by having the patient eat bariums of varied viscosities and meals of varying tastes, textures, and consistencies. E-Z-EM, Inc. created better-tasting barium formulations with varied viscosities in the 1980s in response to vigorous lobbying from speech pathologists. Because it was impractical to have pre-packaged meals impregnated with barium, E-Z-EM developed barium products with uniform texture that mimicked homogenous liquids and solids of varied viscosities (including liquid, nectar, honey, and pudding) to aid in swallowing evaluation.

6.3 DYNAMIC BARIUM SWALLOW PROTOCOL

Many years ago, in 2003, in his seminal book on dysphagia, prof. Olle Ekberg advocated the use of video recorders to tape fluoroscopy sessions during barium swallows, to allow a morphodynamical analysis of the upper GI tract and avoid acquiring 'pointless' static images images. Almost 20 years ago, he was already aware of the impending manometry revolution and of the fact that classic barium radiography was to become of little or no need to the diagnosis. Now, barium swallow exam techniques may differ greatly between institutions. What does not change, though, are the two components of the examination, the first involving the evaluation of the hypopharynx with the cervical esophagus and, subsequently, the assessment of the thoracic esophagus using fluoroscopy or, as in our case, acquisition of frames in cine-modality. Our protocol starts where all protocols should start, no matter what will happen next: history taking and control films. We advise radiologists to carefully take each patient's clinical history before the examination takes place; in our own experience, patients referred to barium swallow for many reasons actually ended up with a suspect diagnosis of achalasia. Taking the clinical history should obviously focus on dysphagia, its duration and onset, asking whether it refers to solids and/or liquids and asking for other symptoms such as those we extensively talked about in Chapter 4, mainly regurgitation, heartburn, and chest pain. A heartfelt advice is to let the patients talk, only interrupting them when their talk goes astray; they usually point out very clearly what is going on with them and this is of invaluable help, concerning the execution and reporting of barium swallows. Another important thing to take care of, before the actual morphodynamical assessment begins, is to acquire control films, especially in patients with history of cervical and thoracic surgery. Good practice requires acquisition of anteroposterior and lateral films of the neck and just anteroposterior of the thorax, which includes the upper abdomen, the latter allowing the assessment of eventual bowel perforations. In patients with dysphagia, we perform the complete dynamic barium swallow, first examining the pharynx and upper esophagus, then mid- and lower esophagus, in double contrast. The single contrast evaluation of pharynx and esophagus starts by positioning the patient in the right lateral position (RL), with the patient's right shoulder close to the detector. The lateral view of the upper esophagus and pharynx should include the top of the palate. We advise to set the magnification to medium, acquiring at six frames per second. Timing is very important: you should start acquiring just as you ask the patient to swallow or just before, stopping as soon as there is maximal distension of the most distal part of the visible esophagus. The AP view of the upper esophagus and pharynx should be taken at the same level craniocaudally as the lateral view, but with tighter coning to produce a narrower image, if you prefer. No change in machine position is required. Magnification should be kept to medium, acquiring at three to four frames per second. Like before, you should start acquiring just as you ask the patient to swallow or just before, stopping as soon as there is maximal distension of the most distal part of the visible esophagus. The middle part of the esophagus is acquired in the right anterior oblique (RAO) position (Figure 6.2), with the patient's right shoulder closer to the detector and facing it, or in the left posterior oblique (LPO) position (Figure 6.3), which is the one we prefer routinely, with the patient giving the back to the detector, left shoulder closer to it. At this point, effervescent tablets or granules should be administered to the patient to obtain double contrast images. Coning should be used laterally to narrow the image as much as possible, without obscuring any of the esophagus, with magnification set at low, acquiring at three frames per second, from

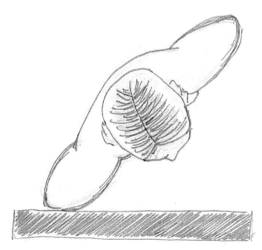

FIGURE 6.2 Scheme of the right anterior oblique projection. Image art courtesy of Simona Borrelli.

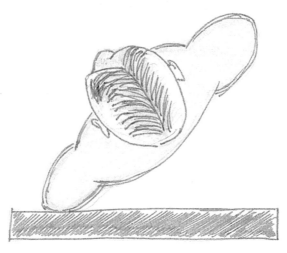

FIGURE 6.3 Scheme of the left posterior oblique projection. Image art courtesy of Simona Borrelli.

the moment the patient is invited to swallow until there is maximal distension of the most distal part of the visible esophagus. The distal esophagus can also be acquired either in the RAO or LPO positions, our group preferring the latter in clinical practice (Figure 6.4). We also prefer to acquire the distal esophagus separately and not in a single run with the middle esophagus, using medium magnification and a number of frames variable from one to three; we tend to use more frames when in need to demonstrate spasm. Start acquiring two seconds after inviting the patient to swallow, stopping just as soon as there is maximal distension of the gastroesophageal junction. Optional frontal acquisition of the lower esophagus may be added, similarly acquired. This protocol should be considered just like some solid foundations on which we can work, but very often it cannot, or should not be carried out exactly as explained, every time. Each patient is different, and we have clearly seen in the previous chapter how especially patients with achalasia tend to fall in one of three phenotypes. The morphodynamical analysis we propose here is something that requires constant attention from the radiologist, who must be present and may even lead the examination in first person. Only by doing this, one might be able to 'tailor' the examination on the single patient, with his or her own peculiar disease. Even during the execution of the exam, the radiologist has to focus the attention on the presence of the five main findings, which as we will see in the next chapter, form the basis of our FBF scoring system: bird-beak sign, endoluminal stasis, esophageal dilation, hypotonia, and spasm. Keeping in mind the manometric considerations of the Chicago Classification, one might be able to recognize, even at first glance, the achalasia phenotype that is being studied, forcing a 'tailored' examination. For example, in a patient that clearly shows a 'classic', hypotonic subtype 1 pattern, with the presence of bird-beak sign, hypotonia, endoluminal stasis with esophageal dilation of varying degree, there is little need of acquiring multiple frames per second, when one or two per second might just be enough; what could be truly helpful in such a case would be to add, or incorporate, a timed barium esophagogram in the protocol, to assess the degree of esophageal emptying at the moment of the diagnosis

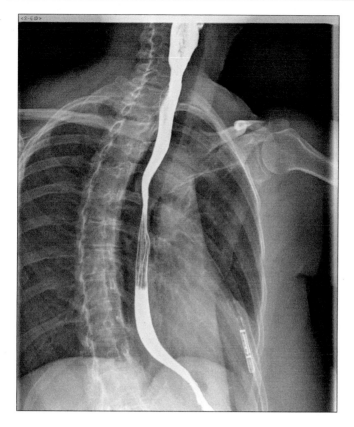

FIGURE 6.4   Esophagus in the LPO projection. LPO and RAO are the best possible projections to avoid superimposition of the thoracic spine.

and, hopefully, to monitor the patient's progress after therapy. When, instead, we recognize subtype 2 or 3 patterns and, more specifically, when there is the need to demonstrate the presence of spasm, one may acquire the mid- and lower esophagus using three to six frames per second. This kind of fluid adapting of the protocol has to become second nature for those practicing barium swallow on a daily basis; moreover, it allows you to have a clear idea of the case and mentally 'report' the examination, making the actual reporting process faster and a mere formality. It is not difficult nor impossible to attain, but it requires study and practice.

6.4 TIMED BARIUM ESOPHAGOGRAM

Barium esophagography and dynamic barium swallow are usually performed to assess the esophagus in a detailed way, both from a morphological and a functional way. The need for a timed barium esophagogram (TBE) arises when we specifically have to study the esophageal emptying, both in the first place at the moment of the diagnosis and, especially after therapy. TBE allows the quantification of the esophageal emptying easily and very accurately. The technique used to obtain TBE is substantially similar to other barium swallow protocols, even though many different techniques to perform TBE have been described in the literature by various authors and with some variations. The protocol we adopt requires using a standard radiography device, not necessarily with cine-acquisition, with the patient, advised to fast overnight before the examination, in the erect posture and in the left posterior oblique position (LPO) or, as we prefer doing, in the frontal view. Multiple films are acquired at fixed time intervals after a single swallow of a specific volume of diluted barium suspension, generally of a specific density. We tend to use low density barium suspensions (45% w/v), asking the patients to ingest a variable volume, generally 100 to 250 ml, in 15–20 seconds. Even though we prefer to use 200 ml as a fixed standard volume in our protocol, to allow a standardized evaluation, especially if the same patient is then reevaluated after therapy, the volume of suspension we may use has to be able to fill the dilated esophagus adequately *and* not harm the patient, causing regurgitation or aspiration. After ingestion is complete, considering barium completely empties from esophagus in one minute in most and in five minutes in all healthy individuals, images are acquired in the left posterior oblique at one, two, and five minutes, generally using three-on-one spot radiographs, or two-on-one spot radiographs when the esophagus is so dilated it would not fit on a smaller radiogram. It is important to keep the distance between patient and the fluoroscope carriage constant through all the examination. While some argue that the two-minute radiograph may be optional, at two-minutes we perform fluoroscopy and acquire a short sequence at a rate of three images per second, to check on the state of esophageal emptying. What can be omitted is the five-minute acquisition, but only when barium has completely cleared from the esophagus on the two-minute film. As we pointed out before, considering TBE usually is performed in sequential studies, before and after treatment for achalasia, to obtain consistent results one should ideally use the same volume of barium in every patient or, at least, in the same patient. It is, therefore, of utmost importance to state the precise amount of barium consumed on the report. By performing the examination in such a fashion, it is possible to assess the degree of esophageal emptying, both qualitatively and quantitatively. To perform a quantitative assessment, one should measure the height of the barium column from its distinct superior level to the gastroesophageal junction, the latter being identified by the classic bird-beak sign in patients with achalasia. The height is quantified by tracing two horizontal parallel lines both at the lowest and at the highest barium level, measuring the distance between them. It is also possible to measure the diameter of the esophagus at the widest point of the barium column found perpendicularly to the long axis of the esophagus. Emptying assessment may be performed by using height and width in sequential images, and eventual post-therapy improvements may be recognized by doing the very same thing on sequential studies. Another method that can be used to assess esophageal emptying, something we prefer doing in our practice, is to calculate the area of the endoluminal barium column at one, two, and five minutes, making a much more precise assessment (Figure 6.5). This is what makes TBE a highly reproducible technique to estimate esophageal emptying,

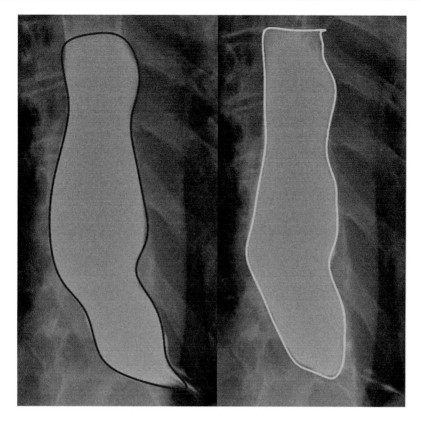

FIGURE 6.5   Timed barium esophagram. Area tracing and comparing.

with an almost perfect inter-observer agreement. There are, however, some small pit-falls to be avoided carefully. Sometimes, the height of the barium column may not fit lengthwise on one film; in this case, a spot film should be acquired centered over the lower portion of esophagus and another image acquired centered over the upper portion of the esophagus. Afterward, a fixed point should be located on each film, generally a vertebral body, serving as a reference point for both images. The barium column shall now be measured both above and below the reference point, on the respective films and the height of the entire barium column obtained by adding the two measurements. The presence of prominent tertiary esophageal contractions in patients with subtype 2 or, especially, subtype 3 achalasia makes it really difficult to acquire images and obtain a continuous barium column. When in this situation, images should be acquired only when the esophagus is relaxed. Retained food material and secretions are often found in achalasia, and these may form a barium-foam interface after barium ingestion and the height of the barium column may be difficult objectively difficult to measure. When in the presence of a barium-foam interface, the superior aspect of the barium column should be measured at a point where the margin is well defined and consistent.

6.5 CLASSIC BARIUM SWALLOW

Of course, it is not possible to carry out the morphodynamical analysis we advocate so strongly in this book, exactly as it should be performed, without the right equipment. Digital direct devices are progressively being implemented, but we are aware that technology improvements, due to costs or 'cultural' problems, often take time to enter routine clinical practice. One way of solving this problem would be, as already stated before and suggested by prof. Ekberg in his seminal work on dysphagia, to equip fluoroscopy with a videotape recorder, or similar digital recording device, allowing fluoroscopy to be recorded every time the pedal is pushed down. This requires very little costs and would allow a morphodynamical examination of the esophagus to be carried out. However, we do understand this is not easy to do and for many different reasons. If there is no way of recording fluoroscopy, all that can be done is a cautious classic 'static' examination, using in-vivo fluoroscopy for dynamical considerations. The protocol we suggest to adopt in these circumstances is a slightly modified version of our morphodynamical evaluation. After control films, lateral and frontal for pharynx and cervical esophagus, just frontal for the thorax, the exam should start in the right lateral position, with a spot film acquired when dilation of cervical esophagus is obtained; fluoroscopy should be used here to assess eventual penetration/aspiration or problems related to 'high' dysphagia. The evaluation of the mid- and lower esophagus should be carried out by acquiring each, on three-on-one radiographs, in the right posterior oblique, frontal, and left posterior oblique views.

6.6 FURTHER READING

Allen BC, Baker ME, Falk GW. Role of barium esophagography in evaluating dysphagia. *Cleve Clin J Med*. 2009;76;105–11.

Baker ME, Einstein DM, Herts BR, et al. Gastroesophageal reflux disease: integrating the barium esophagram before and after antireflux surgery. *Radiology*. 2007;243;329–39.

Chaudhry SR, Bordoni B. *StatPearls* [Internet]. StatPearls Publishing; Treasure Island (FL): Jul 31, 2020. Anatomy, Thorax, Esophagus.

Chung JJ, Park HJ, Yu JS, et al. A comparison of esophagography and esophageal transit scintigraphy in the evaluation of usefulness of endoscopic pneumatic dilatation in achalasia. *Acta Radiol*. 2008;49;498–505.

Debi U, Sharma M, Singh L, Sinha A. Barium esophagogram in various esophageal diseases: a pictorial essay. *Indian J Radiol Imaging*. 2019;29(2):141–54.

de Oliveira JM, Birgisson S, Doinoff C, et al. Timed barium swallow: a simple technique for evaluating esophageal emptying in patients with achalasia. *AJR Am J Roentgenol*. 1997;169;473–9.

Desai JP, Moustarah F. *StatPearls* [Internet]. StatPearls Publishing; Treasure Island (FL): Jun 2, 2020. Esophageal Stricture.

Ghoshal UC, Rangan M. A review of factors predicting outcome of pneumatic dilation in patients with achalasia cardia. *J Neurogastroenterol Motil*. 2011;17;9–13.

Ghoshal UC, Rangan M, Misra A. Pneumatic dilation for achalasia cardia: reduction in lower esophageal sphincter pressure in assessing response and factors associated with recurrence during long-term follow up. *Dig Endosc*. 2012;24;7–15.

Goldenberg SP, Burrell M, Fette GG, Vos C, Traube M. Classic and vigorous achalasia: a comparison of manometric, radiographic, and clinical findings. *Gastroenterology*. 1991;101;743–8.

Gupta M, Ghoshal UC, Verma A, et al. Timed barium esophagogram and high resolution manometry for assessment of response to pneumatic dilation for achalasia cardia: a comparative study [abstract]. *J Gastroenterol Hepatol*. 2012;27;58.

Ishii T, Akaishi T, Abe M, Takayama S, Koseki K, Kamei T, Nakano T. Importance of barium swallow test and chest CT scan for correct diagnosis of achalasia in the primary care setting. *Tohoku J Exp Med*. 2019;247(1):41–9.

Jaffer NM, Ng E, Au FW, Steele CM. Fluoroscopic evaluation of oropharyngeal dysphagia: anatomic, technical, and common etiologic factors. *AJR Am J Roentgenol*. 2015;204(1):49–58.

Kostic SV, Rice TW, Baker ME, et al. Timed barium esophagogram: a simple physiologic assessment for achalasia. *J Thorac Cardiovasc Surg*. 2000;120;935–43.

Levine MS, Rubesin SE. Diseases of the esophagus: diagnosis with esophagography. *Radiology*. 2005;237;414–27.

Neyaz Z, Gupta M, Ghoshal UC. How to perform and interpret timed barium esophagogram. *J Neurogastroenterol Motil*. 2013;19:251–6.

Oezcelik A, Hagen JA, Halls JM, et al. An improved method of assessing esophageal emptying using the timed barium study following surgical myotomy for achalasia. *J Gastrointest Surg*. 2009;13;14–18.

O'Neill OM, Johnston BT, Coleman HG. Achalasia: a review of clinical diagnosis, epidemiology, treatment and outcomes. *World J Gastroenterol*. 2013;19(35):5806–12.

Sanghi V, Thota PN. Barrett's esophagus: novel strategies for screening and surveillance. *Ther Adv Chronic Dis*. 2019;10:2040622319837851.

Vaezi MF, Baker ME, Achkar E, Richter JE. Timed barium oesophagram: better predictor of long term success after pneumatic dilation in achalasia than symptom assessment. *Gut*. 2002;50;765–70.

Vaezi MF, Baker ME, Richter JE. Assessment of esophageal emptying post-pneumatic dilation: use of the timed barium esophagram. *Am J Gastroenterol*. 1999;94;1802–7.

Image Interpretation and FBF Scoring System

Giovanni Fontanella and Simona Borrelli

Contents

7.1 INTRODUCTION

The need for a new, systematic way of approaching, interpreting and reporting barium swallow, especially in patients with achalasia, arises from the fact that we believe that in life and in medicine in particular, there should not be waste of resources, knowledge and time. Too many a time, we have witnessed poorly conducted examinations with subpar reporting. Achalasia may be a rare disease, but a radiologist should always be aware of the possibility of facing a patient with dysphagia and should be fully prepared to

DOI: 10.1201/9781003320302-7

carefully execute and correctly interpret the images. As stated before, the reporting process begins while taking the clinical history, when usually the patient, especially when wisely guided by the physician, points out his or her problems very clearly. The actual reporting does continue while the exam is being executed, with images being interpreted real-time, in vivo, allowing the imaging protocol to be tailored to the specific needs of the patient and, of course, of the radiologist. As we will see, the FBF Scoring System (FBF being the Fatebenefratelli Hospital in Benevento, Italy, where we are based and the scoring system was developed) is not only just a way of prognostically dividing patients in three subtypes, in complete agreement with clinical phenotypes cited in the manometric Chicago Classification; it is rather an organic and systematic pathway that guides the radiologist, using a simple checklist, from image interpretation to structured reporting, avoiding easy mistakes and upgrading the overall quality of the service. The FBF scoring system is the first systematic radiological classification not to be based just on morphology alone, specifically varying degrees of oesophageal dilation, because it integrates dynamic findings with morphological data, making it rather improbable to miss a diagnosis. The most important aspect of the FBF scoring system, in our opinion, is that being completely in agreement with the clinical-manometric Chicago Classification, radiologists, gastroenterologists, surgeons and the rest of the Upper GI MultiDisciplinary Team end up speaking the same 'language', this meaning that a radiology report will be finally something really worth reading and relying upon, a great support to the endoscopic and, especially, manometric diagnoses. At the same time, the simple FBF checklist breaks the image interpretation process down to just five parameters to assess.

7.2 THE FBF CHECKLIST

The FBF checklist, as shown in Table 7.1, is a simple list of five imaging findings, or parameters, that have to be looked for and assessed to correctly diagnose and grade achalasia patients. These findings, namely bird-beak sign, esophageal dilation, hypotonia, endoluminal stasis and spasm, are those to look upon to effectively interpret barium swallow in a patient with achalasia. As we will see in section 7.8, each of these findings is given a specific score, when present. The different combinations of present findings, with the aid of the checklist and scoring system, are efficiently linked to a specific achalasia subtype.

TABLE 7.1 FBF Checklist.

Bird-beak sign
Oesophageal dilation
Hypotonia
Endoluminal stasis
Spasm

7.3 BIRD-BEAK SIGN

The bird-beak sign, sometimes even referred to as 'rat-tail sign' is maybe the best-known and most easily recognisable radiographic sign of achalasia (Figure 7.1). The term bird-beak refers to the shape of the tapered, conical and smooth oesophageal lumen in proximity of the gastro-oesophageal junction, which is significantly narrowed in patients with achalasia. While this sign is common to all three achalasia subtypes, it is more easily recognised in patients with classic, hypotonic subtype 1 achalasia. The involved oesophageal segment is generally 1 to 3 cm long, with smooth mucosal profile, with no sign of abrupt contour changes, local masses nor nodularity; some degree of pliability is retained. Differential diagnosis mainly includes intrinsic or extrinsic malignancies but other conditions, too, such as peptic strictures, Chagas disease, pancreatic pseudocysts and post-surgical complications (especially after fundoplication and vagotomy). Findings suspect for secondary achalasia are many. A tapered segment long at least 3.5 cm or more is highly suspect for regional malignancy, especially cancer of the gastric cardia and esophageal adenocarcinoma. Pseudo- or secondary achalasia are generally characterised by a longer, rigid, asymmetric and irregularly shaped tapering; sometimes, especially in the case of malignancy of the cardia, the involved segment might include the distal esophagus even above the gastro-oesophageal junction. To correctly identify a bird-beak sign, we invite the reporting physician to check the presence of all the items in Table 7.2.

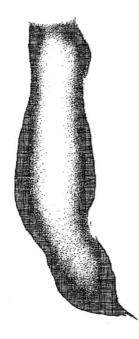

FIGURE 7.1   Post-processed scheme of bird-beak sign.

Source: Image courtesy of Giovanni Fontanella, MD.

TABLE 7.2   Bird-Beak Sign Items.

Smooth, conical tapering
Length of EGJ involved: 1–3 cm
Relatively symmetrical
No nodularity
No signs of local masses

7.4 OESOPHAGEAL DILATION

In 1980, in his seminal work *Gastrointestinal Radiology*, Marcel Brombart described achalasia as a single, progressively deteriorating condition, in which, apart from the classic bird-beak sign, the main factor to consider was lumen dilation, describing four stages of the disease: Stage I, more mild achalasia, diagnosed when lumen caliber measured less than 4 cm; Stage II, or moderate achalasia, in which the caliber of the esophageal lumen measured between 4 and 6 cm; Stage III, or severe achalasia, diagnosed when the caliber measured 6 cm or more. Sigmoid achalasia, in which the overtly dilated, unpropulsive lumen basically folds upon itself, is described as end-stage, or Stage IV achalasia (Figure 7.2). Even considering the relatively recent introduction of the Chicago

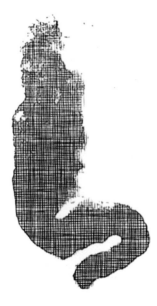

FIGURE 7.2   Post-processed scheme of luminal dilation.

Source: Image courtesy of Giovanni Fontanella, MD.

Classification and all its implications in the clinical practice, these assumptions connecting lumen caliber and dilation with the severity of disease still yield some degree of truth, though especially when considering the evolution of the disease in singularly taken patients and, obviously, in patients with subtype 1, hypotonic achalasia, in which the dilation is more evident than in other subtypes. It is clear, however, that even though esophageal dilation is an important parameter to assess in all patients with achalasia, because it can be present in all subtypes, albeit in varying degrees, it is just one of the many findings that characterises this disease and not the main discriminating factor between different stages. We do integrate Brombart's teachings in our morphodynamical analysis of the achalasic oesophagus by keeping his dimensional staging of dilation in four degrees, as we will see in section 7.8. Oesophageal dilation is present when the caliber is at least 3 cm in diameter, considering the lower axis of the esophagus. To correctly identify and grade esophageal dilation, we invite the reporting physician to check all the items in Table 7.3.

TABLE 7.3 Oesophageal Dilation Grades.

Present when caliber > 3 cm
Grade I: caliber < 4 cm
Grade II: 4 cm < caliber < 6 cm
Grade III: caliber > 6 cm

7.5 VISCERAL HYPOTONIA

Hypotonia or, in some cases, atonia is one of the main radiographic features of achalasia. To be precise, our clinically driven approach to the morphodynamical analysis leads us to the conclusion that hypotonia, defined as absence of apparent oesophageal contractions, with no episodes of panpressurisation or spasms, is actually a typical feature of subtype 1 achalasia, often associated with oesophageal dilation of varying degree. Our definition of hypotonia, deeply based on the Chicago Classification pathophysiologic assumptions, if kept in mind when reviewing dynamical barium swallow series, effectively enables the reporting physician to diagnose subtype 1 achalasia, ruling out subtypes 2 and 3. Rather than assessing hypotonia, what we do is actually assessing oesophageal motility to recognise the exact motility pattern in the specific patient. At the same time, as we will see in section 7.7, while the presence of spasm effectively rules out subtypes 1 and 2, the absence of both hypotonia and spasms rules out subtypes 1 and 3, configuring the presence of a subtype 2, in which panpressurisation is evident, with tertiary, unpropulsive waves. This is, in our opinion, the most important pattern to be analysed, the true essence of morphodynamic imaging in achalasia; to effectively accomplish this assessment, a thorough knowledge of pathophysiology (Chapter 4) and a basic grasp of manometry (Chapter 5, section 4) are needed. To correctly identify oesophageal hypotonia, we invite the reporting physician to check all the items in Table 7.4.

TABLE 7.4　Hypotonia.

No apparent contractions
No panpressurisation
No spasms

7.6 ENDOLUMINAL STASIS

Considering the intrinsic nature of achalasia, another important radiologic hallmark of all forms of the disease is endoluminal stasis (Figure 7.3). There are many ways to accomplish the assessment of barium stasis in the oesophageal lumen. One way of doing this is, of course, by using a timed barium esophagogram by acquiring images after the patient ingests a 200 ml bolus in 15–20 seconds, at one, two, and five minutes, subsequently tracing the upper barium level in all three images, comparing them. We tend to use this method of assessing stasis only in patients who are to undergo pneumatic dilation, or other surgical/endoscopic treatment, because it allows an effective and precise quantification of the oesophageal emptying, too, enabling a comparison between pre- and post-treatment images, to check on, and quantify, eventual improvements. Now, the presence of endoluminal stasis is generally very evident, even during the execution of the exam; to allow correct reporting, though, efficient diagnostic criteria are needed. To assess endoluminal stasis, during the examination and after at least two boluses are ingested, we invite the patient to ingest another consistent barium bolus, a test bolus, after making sure the current barium level is under the aortic portion of the oesophagus; we then proceed to acquire two short series of the same length, usually two or three seconds, three images per second, at one and five minutes after ingestion, considering that at five minutes, the oesophagus should be clear of endoluminal content in healthy individuals. Upper barium levels are traced and compared as explained in Chapter 6, section 4 (Figure 7.4). Barium stasis is confirmed when the heights of the barium columns are comparable (with a tolerance margin of 10 mm). Another way of comparing evaluations at one and five minutes might be, as shown in the images, by tracing and calculating the areas occupied by barium. To correctly identify endoluminal stasis, we invite the reporting physician to check all the items in Table 7.5.

TABLE 7.5　Endoluminal Stasis.

Evaluation at 1 and 5 mins after test bolus
Comparable height of barium columns (+– 10 mm)
No spasms

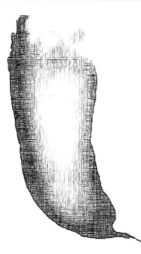

FIGURE 7.3 Post-processed scheme of endoluminal stasis.

Source: Image courtesy of Giovanni Fontanella, MD.

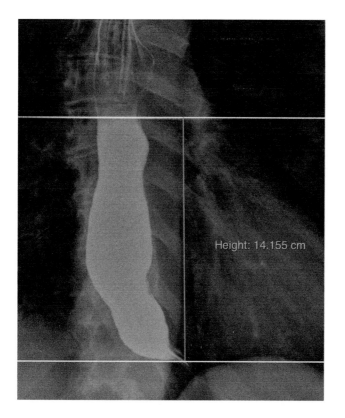

FIGURE 7.4 Measurement of barium column height in timed barium esophagram.

7.7 SPASM

The presence of spasm is practically pathognomonic for subtype 3 patients, just as the presence of hypotonia/atonia is typical in subtype 1 patients. Spasm is easily detected at the morphodynamical assessment, usually in a radiographic imaging pattern already very suggestive for subtype 3, previously known as vigorous achalasia. What we intend for spasm should not to be mistaken for the tertiary, uncoordinated, and unpropulsive waves typical of (but not exclusive to) the panpressurising subtype 2 and present in the whole of the oesophagus; it is rather the product of impaired relaxation of the LES plus active spastic contractions of the mid- and distal oesophagus that translate into what is known as a corkscrew pattern, an irregular succession of massively narrow and dilated oesophageal portions. This is what differentiates pressure disorders in subtypes 2 and 3; they are both unpropulsive, but in subtype 2, we witness a rather moderately dilated lumen with sporadical tertiary waves and pressurisation, not a succession of narrowed and dilated lumen, typical of subtype 3. This characteristic, spastic pattern is what, most probably, makes subtype 3 the least susceptible to treatment. Moreover, the presence of spasm is often associated with the presence of pseudodiverticula, especially epiphrenic; in achalasia, this happens almost invariably in subtype 3 patients. To correctly identify spasm, we invite the reporting physician to check all the items in Table 7.6.

TABLE 7.6   Spasm.

Mid-, lower oesophagus, LES involved
Corkscrew pattern
No spasms

7.8 FBF SCORING SYSTEM

Our scoring system, named after the institution in which it was developed, the Fatebenefratelli Hospital in Benevento, Italy, should not be considered just a mere tool to obtain patient stratification; even though that was the main aim, when first implemented into our clinical practice, its use prompted the development of the checklist we have gone through in the last few pages and, subsequently, almost inadvertently it helped form the basis for a new, clinically oriented structured reporting form, which will be discussed in detail in Chapter 8. After a period of empiric observation, we concluded that, to obtain an effective radiographic profiling that reflected the new advances of pathophysiology, only five findings (or parameters) were to be focused on (Table 7.7).

Of these parameters, one, namely the bird-beak sign, is in common to all achalasia subtypes and is somewhat pathognomonic, allowing the disease to be radiographically

TABLE 7.7   How to Identify Achalasia Using the FBF Scoring System.

Is the bird-beak sign present?
Is oesophageal dilation present? (if so, measure it)
Is hypotonia/atonia present?
Is endoluminal barium stasis present?
Is spasm of the mid- and lower oesophagus present?

recognised; some others might be in common to the different subtypes, albeit in varying degrees, such as dilation and endoluminal stasis. In the end, we have the two remaining findings on complete opposite sides: hypotonia, typical of atonic subtype 1 achalasia and spasm, typical of spastic, also known as 'vigorous' subtype 3 achalasia. This made the search for a finding or parameter characterising subtype 2 rather useless or even confusing, at worst. The scoring system has been developed as a series of questions to be answered while analysing the morphodynamical examination that leads to diagnosis confirmation and patient stratification. A variable number of points is awarded to each question when positively answered; at the end of the questionary, points are summed up and the final result will position the patient exactly in his or her subtype. Of course, this final result will be a great support to the manometric and endoscopic diagnosis, allowing the radiologist, for the first time, to give pathophysiologic information to the clinician and not just a mere and pointless morphological description of images. Our aim when developing this scoring system was to train the mind of the radiologist to think and critically elaborate the images, to internalise the whole morphodynamical diagnostic process. After all these chapters, tables and images, the specific achalasia subtype that is being analysed should be pretty clear to the eye of the reporting operator, even without a supporting scoring system. Considering many diagnoses of achalasia are still missed to this very day, though, especially in the case of subtype 2 or 3 (because they do not necessarily reflect the 'typical' achalasia findings trainees are taught to look for), a scoring system such as ours was created to serve as a guide, especially for the less expert observer and an easily readable support for the clinician. Many of the findings, namely bird-beak sign, stasis, hypotonia and dilation < 4 cm are given 2 points each, when present; the only exceptions being spasm, awarded −2 points and the higher degrees of dilation have been given 4, between 4 and 6 cm and 6 points, when caliber is > 6 cm (Table 7.8).

Now, summing up all the points in each patient, all the possible combinations will lead to one of three subtypes, which are perfectly comparable to the Chicago Classification subtypes:

- Subtype 1, when the score is 8 or higher;
- Subtype 2, when the score is 6 or 8 (when hypotonia is present, score 8 should be considered subtype 1);
- Subtype 3, when the score is from 0 to 6 (when spasm is present, score 6 should be considered subtype 3).

TABLE 7.8   Findings and Their Relative Scores.

FINDING	POINTS
Bird-beak sign	2
Oesophageal dilation	Ø < 4 cm = 2
	Ø 4–6 cm = 4
	Ø > 6 cm = 6
Endoluminal stasis	2
Hypotonia	2
Spasm	−2

TABLE 7.9   Chicago and FBF's Subtypes Comparison. Score 6 with Spasm Is Subtype III. Score 8 with Hypotonia Is Subtype I.

CHICAGO/FBF SUBTYPE	FBF SCORE
I	8 or > 8
II	6–8
III	0–6

As you might have noticed, this scoring system and our overall approach to achalasia is very much clinically and pathophysiologically oriented; the scoring system was developed drastically separate the 'extreme' subtypes, 1 and 3, obtaining the same, by consequence, for what stays in the middle, subtype 2. Apart from the patient stratification implications that could help communicate with clinicians and surgeons, we reckon the whole approach and checklist should be adopted as a modus operandi for the reporting of achalasia, a process that starts during the execution of the exam (Table 7.9).

7.9 FURTHER READING

Bredenoord AJ, Fox M, Kahrilas PJ, et al. Chicago classification criteria of esophageal motility disorders defined in high resolution esophageal pressure topography. *Neurogastroenterol Motil.* 2012;24(Suppl 1):57–65.

Chen HW, Du M. Minimally invasive surgery for esophageal achalasia. *J Thorac Dis.* 2016;8(7):1834–6.

Clayton SB, Patel R, Richter JE. Functional and anatomic esophagogastric junction outflow obstruction: manometry, timed barium esophagram findings, and treatment outcomes. *Clin Gastroenterol Hepatol.* 2016;14:907–11.

de Oliveira JM, Birgisson S, Doinoff C, et al. Timed barium swallow: a simple technique for evaluating esophageal emptying in patients with achalasia. *AJR Am J Roentgenol.* 1997;169:473–9.

Fontanella G, et al. A proposal for a new prognostic grading system in achalasia using dynamic barium swallow: the FBF score. *EMJ Radiol.* 2021;2(1):34–6.

Goldblum JR, Whyte RI, Orringer MB, Appelman HD. Achalasia: a morphologic study of 42 resected specimens. *Am J Surg Pathol*. 1994;18(4):327–37.

Kostic S, Andersson M, Hellstrom M, et al. Timed barium esophagogram in the assessment of patients with achalasia: reproducibility and observer variation. *Dis Esophagus*. 2005;18:96–103.

Nicodeme F, de Ruigh A, Xiao Y, et al. A comparison of symptom severity and bolus retention with Chicago classification esophageal pressure topography metrics in patients with achalasia. *Clin Gastroenterol Hepatol*. 2013;11:131–7.

Pandolfino JE, Gawron AJ. Achalasia: a systematic review. *JAMA*. 2015;313(18):1841–52.

Rohof WO, Hirsch DP, Kessing BF, et al. Efficacy of treatment for patients with achalasia depends on the distensibility of the esophagogastric junction. *Gastroenterology*. 2012;143:328–35.

Rohof WO, Lei A, Boeckxstaens GE. Esophageal stasis on a timed barium esophagogram predicts recurrent symptoms in patients with long-standing achalasia. *Am J Gastroenterol*. 2013;108:49–55.

Sackett DL, Haynes RB. The architecture of diagnostic research. *Br Med J*. 2002;324:539–41.

Vaezi MF, Baker ME, Achkar E, et al. Timed barium oesophagram: better predictor of long term success after pneumatic dilation in achalasia than symptom assessment. *Gut*. 2002;50:765–70.

Vaezi MF, Baker ME, Richter JE. Assessment of esophageal emptying post-pneumatic dilation: use of the timed barium esophagram. *Am J Gastroenterol*. 1999;94:1802–7.

Structured Reporting

Giovanni Fontanella

Contents

8.1 INTRODUCTION

Prose reporting has been the primary, and for many decades, the only product of radiology since its inception in the early 1900s. It has gone through huge leaps forward in both imaging and reporting technology. However, even though it can be suggested that this is the very reason radiologists should think about updating their reporting practices, it is an undeniable fact that prose reports are intrinsically woven into the profession of the radiologist. One can say, actually, that prose reporting is part of the peculiar value, the unique effort a given radiologist usually brings to his or her practice of medicine; at the same time, this causes strong resistance to standardisation, especially among radiologists of older generations. An important study from Johnson et al., evaluating structured-reporting systems against traditional, free-text dictation, for this very reason explicitly excluded older radiologists, assuming their intrinsic preference for prose reporting. When thinking of implementing structured reporting, an apparently easy task, one might have to fight this peculiar form of resistance to change. It should be noted that, as in life, the only constant in the profession of the radiologist and radiology itself should be change and adaptability to change, because this specific medical branch is still very young and has evolved exponentially, going from Röntgen to radiomics in a little more than 100 years. Truth is, however, we need not change just for the sake of it; we need it when we feel it brings us something more than we already have, when it gives us tools to simplify our practices, to quicken and standardise the diagnostic process. This last concept, 'standardisation', is what actually scares narrow-minded radiologists

DOI: 10.1201/9781003320302-8

the most, because it is often mistaken for a will to dehumanise the reporting process; it is, of course, not what we intend to do. At the same time, while we strongly advocate the use of structured reporting for barium swallow examinations in patients with oesophageal motility disorders, we recognise that not every kind of examination might benefit from a schematic way of interpreting and reporting images, as the already cited study from Johnson et al. suggests. Barium swallows, and especially the way we perform barium swallows, yield such a diverse wealth of diagnostic and prognostic information that prose reporting might dangerously result in decreases in accuracy and completeness— that, and no other, is the main reason we use our specifically developed structured template and advise its adoption. Our structured template is based on the assumption that checklist-based medical practice has shown to be safer, more efficient and consistent, highly reproducible and standardisable. A wider adoption of such way of reporting and executing exams would allow for a quick, precise, prognostically and therapeutically oriented diagnosis anywhere in the world, not just in our institution.

8.2 CHECKLIST-BASED REPORTING

Albeit treated separately in a dedicated chapter, the checklist-based reporting process is to be considered seamlessly integrated into the single mental effort the radiologist has to make while acquiring and reviewing the examination. The mere act of reporting should be just a bureaucratic formality to be tackled at the end of the whole procedure. Considering the aim of the radiologist interested in oesophageal imaging should be that of quickly identifying the disease or disease spectrum, or rather exclude a disease or disease spectrum, trying to give the clinician as much morphodynamical data as possible. Our proposed checklist-based reporting is a clean, fast and reproducible way of doing this; we advocate its use not only in patients with suspected achalasia spectrum disease, but in every patient with suspected oesophageal motility disorder, as its schematic clarity allows the observer to quickly and exactly point out what is wrong with the observed motility pattern. All these assumptions have been condensed into a schematic fill-in form, in which the five cardinal findings, described in Chapter 7, are assessed for presence and severity; an FBF score can be then quickly calculated and the patient's suspected achalasia subtype pointed out (Figure 8.1). Of course, this checklist was developed with achalasia spectrum diseases, so the first finding we suggest looking out for is the pathognomonic bird-beak sign, by which we refer, it is worth repeating ourselves, to the shape of the tapered, conical and smooth oesophageal lumen in proximity of the gastro-oesophageal junction, significantly narrowed in patients with achalasia and clear sign of GEJ impairment. While this sign is common to all three achalasia subtypes, please bear in mind that it is more easily recognised in patients with classic, hypotonic subtype 1 achalasia. The presence of a bird-beak sign, which sometimes has to be carefully searched for in the dynamic series, as it might often times be not as evident or quickly disappearing, is strongly suggestive of a GEJ impairment connected to primary achalasia, especially when the involved oesophageal segment is

Xxx Medical Center

Reason for Study: Dysphagia, suspected achalasia

Referring Physician: Dr. Wick, John

Evaluating Clinician: Fontanella, Giovanni.   Patient ID: xx Study Number: xx
Patient Name: Status: Inpatient
Age: Gender: Male
Height: xx kgs - Current Weight: xx cms - Body Mass Index: xx

ITEM DESCRIPTOR	SCORE	GUIDE	COMMENT	PREVIOUS SCORE
Bird-beak sign		Specify bird-beak sign type. If transient, specify sequence and frame in which it is detected.	xx bird-beak type.	xx bird-beak type.
Dilation		Specify dilation grade. Grade I = 3<x<4 cm (2 points); Grade II = 4<x<6 cm (4 points); Grade III = >6 cm (6 points)	Dilation Grade: Dilation Score:	Dilation Grade: Dilation Score
Hypotonia		Specify whether present or not. Specify whether hypotonia or atonia is present.		
Stasis		Calculate stasis at time 0 (onset), 2, 5 and 10 minutes. Two points when present from time 2 minutes on.	Column height: - Time 0: - 2 minutes: - 5 minutes: - 10 minutes: - Custom:	Column height: - Time 0: - 2 minutes: - 5 minutes: - 10 minutes: - Custom:
Spasm		Specify whether present and in which portions. -2 points when present.	Present from oesophageal portion x to portion x.	Present from oesophageal portion x to portion x.
FBFs		ACHALASIA TYPE I = 8-12 POINTS ACHALASIA TYPE II = 6-8 POINTS ACHALASIA TYPE III = 0-6 POINTS When hypotonia is present, score 8 is to be considered type I. When spasm is present, score 6 is to be considered type III.		

FIGURE 8.1 FBF-based structured reporting format.

generally 1 to 3 cm long, with a smooth mucosal profile and no sign of abrupt contour changes, local masses or nodularity. A present bird-beak sign is worth 2 FBF score points; if no bird-beak sign is found, after careful examination, primary achalasia spectrum diseases can be ruled out, unless the patient has already been manometrically diagnosed with GEJ impairment, as it might happen that the GEJ is so tight that little or no barium enters the lumen. In this case, however, we strongly suggest referring the patient to upper GI endoscopy to rule out secondary disease. The second item we need to check while reviewing a morphodynamical examination of the oesophagus, is lumen dilation. Our form allows the observer to check the presence and severity of lumen dilation, which might be present in all three achalasia subtypes but is, as already stated, the hallmark of hypotonic/atonic subtype 1 achalasia. We included Brombart's dimensional staging into our severity evaluation of oesophageal dilation, both as a tribute and because its prognostic implications, albeit in subtype 1 achalasia only, are still valid. As we already know, we consider a luminal caliber to be normal, measuring on the short axis of the oesophagus, when it is 3 cm or less. Dilation is therefore deemed as present when the caliber is at least 3 cm in width. After presence is confirmed, severity is assessed by attributing the appropriate amount of FBF score points: 2 points if the caliber measures less than 4 cm, 4 points if the caliber stands between 4 and 6 cm, 6 points if the caliber measures more than 6 cm. The third item to be checked is endoluminal stasis of the barium bolus. As already explained in Chapter 6, section 4, the presence of endoluminal stasis is detected by using the timed barium esophagogram technique, tracing and comparing the upper level on a frontally acquired series at one and five minutes after ingestion of a fixed amount of barium suspension—we suggest using 200 ml as a fixed amount in all patients, to allow for reproducibility and comparability; the usage of a same, custom amount of barium suspension in the same patient, in time, is mandatory, because it allows to detect improving or deteriorating conditions, or quantify post-surgical/post-dilation improvements. Barium levels at one and five minutes are deemed comparable when the height of the second measurement differs less than 10 mm from the first. The presence of endoluminal stasis can be detected in all three types of achalasia, but it is more commonly found in types I and II, due to the severely reduced or impaired peristalsis. The checklist assessment ends with the evaluation of oesophageal peristalsis. While assessing a patient with achalasia, even though this might apply to all patients with oesophageal motility diseases, one might find three possible scenarios: atonic/severely hypotonic, dystonic or spasmodic disturbs. In the case of achalasia, the evidence afinalistic non-propulsive or, in severe cases, absent peristalsis, usually coupled with lumen dilation and endoluminal stasis, clearly depicts classic, type I achalasia; this is awarded with 2 FBF score points. Tertiary, spasmodic peristalsis, configuring a 'rosary bead' or 'corkscrew' appearance of the oesophagus, especially involving the distal two-thirds of the viscer, strongly suggests the presence of a type III achalasia—this is awarded with −2 FBF score points. What stands in between, neither hypotonic/atonic nor spasmodic, is the dystonic panpressurised type II achalasia oesophagus, with the presence of multiple tertiary waves throughout the body of the oesophagus—this is awarded with no FBF score points, as the absence of both hypotonia and spasms effectively rules out type I and III achalasia, configuring a type II.

8.3 FURTHER READING

Al-Hawary MM, Francis IR, Chari ST, et al. Pancreatic ductal adenocarcinoma radiology reporting template: Consensus statement of the Society of Abdominal Radiology and the American Pancreatic Association. *Radiology*. 2014;270:248–60.

Ash JS, Berg M, Coiera E. Some unintended consequences of information technology in health care: The nature of patient care information system-related errors. *J Am Med Inform Assoc*. 2004;11:104–12.

Bosmans JML, Peremans L, Menni M, et al. Structured reporting: If, why, when, how—and at what expense? Results of a focus group meeting of radiology professionals from eight countries. *Insights Imaging*. 2012;3:295–302.

Buntin MB, Jain SH, Blumenthal D. Health information technology: Laying the infrastructure for national health reform. *Health Aff (Millwood)*. 2010;29:1214–19.

Eisenberg RL, Bankier AA, Boiselle PM. Compliance with Fleischner Society guidelines for management of small lung nodules: A survey of 834 radiologists. *Radiology*. 2010;255:218–24.

Gawande A. *The checklist manifesto: How to get things right*. New York: Metropolitan Books; 2010

Hawkins CM, Hall S, Hardin J, et al. Prepopulated radiology report templates: A prospective analysis of error rate and turnaround time. *J Digit Imaging*. 2012;25:504–11.

Johnson AJ, Chen MYM, Swan JS, et al. Cohort study of structured reporting compared with conventional dictation. *Radiology*. 2009;253:74–80.

Kahn CE, Heilbrun ME, Applegate KE. From guidelines to practice: How reporting templates promote the use of radiology practice guidelines. *J Am Coll Radiol*. 2013;10:268–73.

Langlotz CP. Structured radiology reporting: Are we there yet? *Radiology*. 2009;253:23–5.

Prevedello LM, Farkas C, Ip IK, et al. Large-scale automated assessment of radiologist adherence to the physician quality reporting system for stroke. *J Am Coll Radiol*. 2012;9:414–20.

Schwartz LH, Panicek DM, Berk AR, et al. Improving communication of diagnostic radiology findings through structured reporting. *Radiology*. 2011;260:174–81.

Sistrom CL, Honeyman-Buck J. Free text versus structured format: Information transfer efficiency of radiology reports. *AJR Am J Roentgenol*. 2005;185:804–12.

Pictorial Essay

9

Giovanni Fontanella

Contents

DOI: 10.1201/9781003320302-9

INTRODUCTION

It goes without saying that proficient learning does actually require physical presence and some degree of face-to-face engagement and discussion. In the case of upper GI morphodynamic imaging, this factor becomes even more crucial. In our experience, while reading some seminal volumes on the matter, especially the writings of prof. Olle Ekberg, which have been both formative and informative, the actual learning took place in dark X-ray practices both at St. Mark's Hospital in London and at the Old Polyclinic Hospital in Naples. While writing these words, we are fully aware that what we are trying to achieve is to pass on information, our experience and love for this branch of imaging, via the written, not spoken word—a rather complex thing to do. The fact that we are actually referring to diagnoses made by observing moving images makes our aim even more difficult, because we will be using and describing still images. In the next pages, we are going to introduce a sign-based pictorial essay, dedicated to each of the five cardinal radiologic signs of achalasia, which will be treated separately. Each image presented hereby will be singularly annotated and commented. We preferred this approach, rather than a case-based, integrated one, because we deemed a sign-based approach to be more didactically valid and much more resemblant of the actual morphodynamical analysis we perform. When analyzing patients with suspected achalasia, our approach to reporting is the step-by-step, sign-by-sign approach we described in the previous chapter, when we introduced our checklist-based structured reporting. As we will see, while some signs such as dilation or spasm can be clearly, or at least more easily demonstrated, even on static images, some others and especially the bird-beak sign might present with some degree of difficulty of detection; a thorough, dedicated series of annotated images for each sign, complete with tips, suggestions and, last but not least, clinical history in the cases we deemed it necessary is, in our opinion, a rather obligatory training to undergo before approaching this kind of patients.

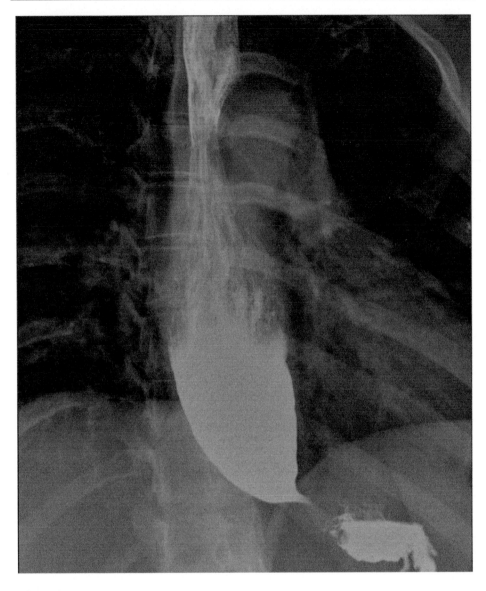

FIGURE 9.1

Clinical Information: 52-year-old man with long-standing clinical history of dysphagia, regurgitation, heartburn, cough and occasional pain after swallowing.

Comment: As we have seen up until this point, achalasia is the direct result of a tight closure of the lower esophageal sphincter; this translates radiologically as the bird-beak sign. Being the first radiologic sign we look for in morphodynamical imaging, it is worth remembering the actual definition of this sign: it is *a smooth, conical, sometimes linear or thin, symmetrical tapering of the gastro-oesophageal junction, with a length between 1 and 3 centimetres, with no sign of nodularity or focal pathology.* A classic, textbook bird-beak sign can be seen in Figure 9.1, as a symmetrical, triangular-conical narrowing of the gastro-oesophageal junction, with a length of less than 3 centimetres. No sign of focal disease can be detected. While the occasional opening of the GEJ lets some of the barium pass into the gastric lumen, the vast majority of the endoluminal contrast stays above the closed GEJ. The presence and correct identification of a bird-beak sign alone is highly suggestive for a diagnosis of achalasia; that is why, in the morphodynamical analysis of patients with suspected achalasia, we look for a tight closure of the GEJ first. In this specific case, the sign is well noted and evident by itself, but it can, in general, be more or less perceptible depending on the degree of tightness of the GEJ. Another important factor that makes this sign more or less apparent is the presence of other suspect findings, which might help in pointing our eyes towards the GEJ: in Figure 9.1, in fact, hypotonia and lumen dilation of medium severity are noted, along a bird-beak sign. A timed barium oesophagram acquired later in the examination pointed out the presence of stasis as well.

Additional Findings: Irritation of the oesophageal mucosal profile at the cardiac portion is noted.

FBF Score and Staging: Bird-beak sign (+), Dilation (++), Hypotonia (+), Stasis (+), Spasm (–) = FBFs 10—type I Achalasia.

Tips: Carefully examine the stack of images on each sequence you acquire. In this case, the bird-beak sign was evident throughout all the examination, but sometimes it can be evident on just one image—*use six to eight frames per second while acquiring on the LES.*

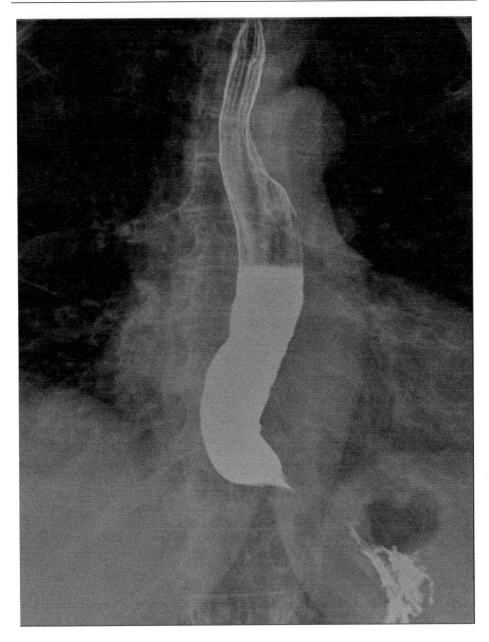

FIGURE 9.2

Clinical Information: 43-year-old obese woman, with clinical history of recent weight loss, solid-prevalent dysphagia, heartburn and occasional regurgitation.

Comment: In this patient, the first clinical suspect was actually oesophageal cancer, but signs of focal disease were not noted. Figure 9.2 elegantly demonstrates the presence of a bird-beak sign but, in truth, the sign was evident on just a couple of frames in this AP sequence: we had to look for it. As we said in the comment to the previous image, the presence of other suspect findings, as a general rule, points our eyes towards the GEJ when we do not do it ourselves. In this case, the other striking findings were stasis and the consequent hypotonia, which we found at the five-minute timed barium acquisition. Subtle bird-beak sign and low-degree dilation were subsequently noted. Morphodynamic imaging saved the day in this case: a static examination might have easily passed as negative.

Additional Findings: Remaining oesophagus is unremarkable. Intimal sclerosis at the aortic arch.

FBF Score and Staging: Bird-beak sign (+), Dilation (+), Hypotonia (+), Stasis (+), Spasm (–) = FBFs 8—type I Achalasia—*please note that Score 8 with Hypotonia is considered type I.*

Tips: As stated before, it is crucial to examine the LES in multiple projections, using at least six to eight frames per second while acquiring, carefully looking for the diverse array of signs in each acquired stack of frames. *It is not unlikely for the bird-beak sign not to be apparent straight away*, so if you suspect achalasia and the examination has been properly carried out, keep searching for it and you will eventually find it.

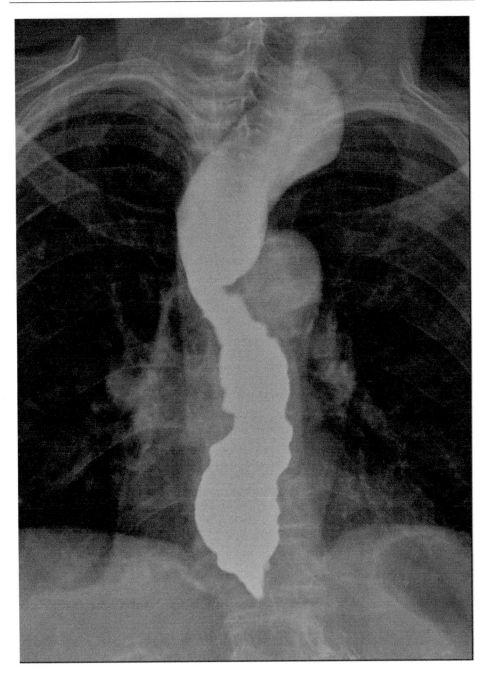

FIGURE 9.3

Clinical Information: 47-year-old woman with a clinical history of dysphagia, odynophagia, regurgitation and heartburn.

Comment: The commonly used definition for this sign, 'bird-beak', might lead sometimes to confusion as to whether the sign is present or not. While the two previous cases were more easily detectable as bird beaks, in this specific case shown in Figure 9.3, the tightly closed GEJ, together with the peculiar panpressurized state of the oesophageal lumen, combine to create a symmetrical, regular, conical image that is, in this case, our bird-beak sign. Our definition of the sign, appropriately enough, is purposely omni-comprehensive to welcome any type of GEJ closure/tightness in it.

Additional Findings: Dilation of medium severity (4.2 cm), irregular panpressurization, between the cardiac portion of the oesophagus and the GEJ, are noted. Stasis was present at the five-minute timed barium control film.

FBF Score and Staging: Bird-beak sign (+), Dilation (++), Hypotonia (−), Stasis (+), Spasm (−) = FBFs 8—type II Achalasia.

Tips: Even though a 'conical' bird-beak sign can be found in all three types of achalasia, because of the specific, pathologic panpressurizing pattern found in the lower two-thirds of the oesophagus, *it is much more common to find such sign morphology in patients with type II achalasia*; this piece of information could be useful to avoid confusion as to whether the sign is present or not in this kind of patients, because of the 'conical' bird beak.

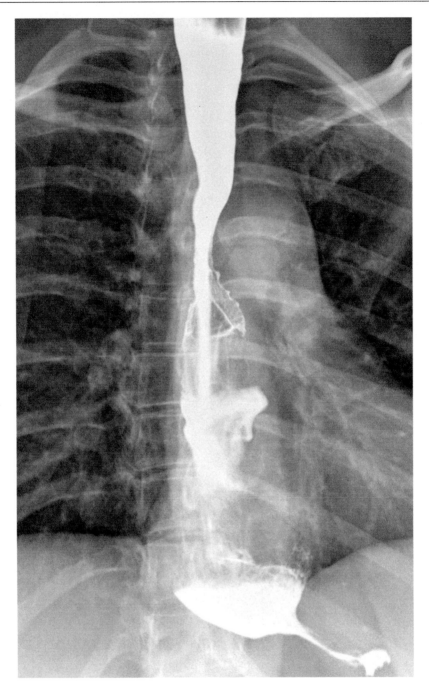

FIGURE 9.4

Clinical Information: 62-year-old man with long-standing clinical history of untreated odynophagia, regurgitation, heartburn and weight loss.

Comment: In Figure 9.4, a rather elongated (3 cm), symmetrical and regular GEJ is noted. It is worth remembering that the sign known as 'bird-beak sign', a locution we conventionally used and will continue to use both in this volume and our clinical activity to avoid confusion, is known by several other names, one of which is 'rat-tail sign'—this definition probably suits the GEJ in Figure 9.4 better. This peculiar configuration has the same clinical meaning of classic bird-beak signs, because it is the radiological translation of an area of high, homogeneous pressure at the LES and should be treated as such.

Additional Findings: Dilation of medium degree, atonia and endoluminal barium stasis at the five-minute control film were all noted.

FBF Score and Staging: Bird-beak sign (+), Dilation (++), Hypotonia (+), Stasis (+), Spasm (–) = FBFs 10—type I Achalasia.

Tips: This elongated bird-beak or 'rat-tail sign' is generally found when the affected portion of the LES is quite long—in this case, 3 cm. This form of the sign can be found in all three types of achalasia, but it is generally associated with type I, atonic achalasia. In fact, in type I patients, the longer the portion of the affected LES, the worse the loss of parietal tone of the oesophageal body. Another problem, aside from the issue of the interpretation of the actual finding, might be that, in some cases, *tumours of the LES with little or no sign of nodularity can present with the very same features*, including the atonic pseudo-achalasia. Even though most patients with suspected achalasia undergo prudential EGD, *in cases such as the one in Figure 9.4, especially when weight loss is noted in clinical history, we deem an EGD to be mandatory and the diagnosis be considered a suspect pseudo-achalasia until otherwise proven.*

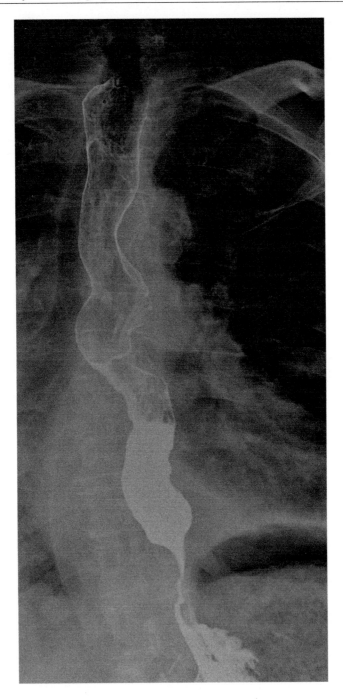

FIGURE 9.5

Clinical Information: 53-year-old woman with a clinical history of dysphagia, chest pain and occasional regurgitation.

Comment: The sign showed in Figure 9.5 can be seen as something in between a classic and a conical bird-beak sign. A symmetric, well-defined, triangularly shaped bird-beak sign might be the result of panpressurization of the lower two-thirds of the oesophageal body and generally, albeit not exclusively, found in patients with type II achalasia.

Additional Findings: Dilation of low severity (3.9 cm), irregular panpressurization, between the cardiac portion of the oesophagus and the GEJ, are noted. Stasis was present at the five-minute timed barium control film.

FBF Score and Staging: Bird-beak sign (+), Dilation (+), Hypotonia (–), Stasis (+), Spasm (–) = FBFs 6—type II Achalasia.

Tips: As for the conical bird-beak sign, this triangular sign is generally associated with panpressurization of the lower two-thirds of the oesophageal body and this combination can be often spotted together from the beginning of the examination and prompt a quick recognition of a type II pattern, even before an FBF score is obtained.

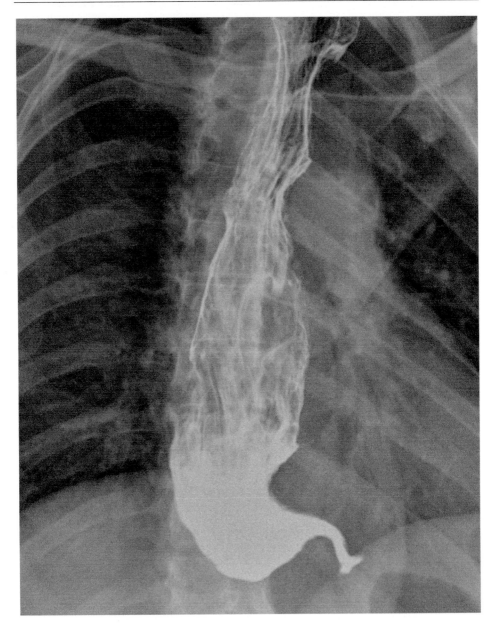

FIGURE 9.6

Clinical Information: 50-year-old woman with long-standing clinical history of dysphagia/odynophagia, regurgitation, heartburn and cough. *Patient specifies she helps herself to plenty of water during meals to reach GEJ opening and partial oesophageal emptying.*

Comment: In a few cases, the GEJ is so tight that, even many minutes after the ingestion of the first barium bolus, it can be difficult to obtain a radiologic demonstration of this tightness, with no bird-beak sign and barium impaction in the oesophageal body—at the same time, it is plainly clear we are observing a pathologic oesophagus suspect for achalasia. In such instances, to demonstrate the GEJ and generally at the end of the examination, when other suggestive signs for achalasia are noted already, except for the bird-beak sign, we use a trick patients themselves use to force the GEJ open: we give them a glass of water to drink. The weight of water, mixed with the already present, generally thick barium in the oesophageal lumen, alters endoluminal pressure to a point that the GEJ opens to the patients' relief. The frame shown in Figure 9.6 clearly shows the moment the GEJ opens to allow some barium in the gastric fundus, 11 minutes after the start of the examination—please note there is no barium in the stomach and that the GEJ is of the elongated form that, as we stated before, is generally, albeit not exclusively, associated with hypo/atonic achalasia, as in this case.

Additional Findings: Dilation of high severity (6.1 cm), atonia, are noted. Stasis was present at the five- and ten-minute timed barium control films.

FBF Score and Staging: Bird-beak sign (+), Dilation (+++), Hypotonia (+), Stasis (+), Spasm (−) = FBFs 12—type I Achalasia.

Tips: Gastro-oesophageal junctions that seldom open spontaneously are frequent in all types of late-stage disease; however, these tend to be more common in types I and II achalasia. The initial absence of a bird-beak sign, when other suggestive signs are present, shall be considered suspect for late-stage disease and prompt provocative manoeuvres, such as drinking water to alter endoluminal pressure and force the GEJ open; as an alternative, one might use the provocative manoeuvre used by the patient during meals, if applicable (carbonated drinks, bread, etc.). We tend to prefer water and generally perform such manoeuvres at the end of the examination, after the other typical signs are clearly noted and five- and ten-minute timed barium control films have already been acquired.

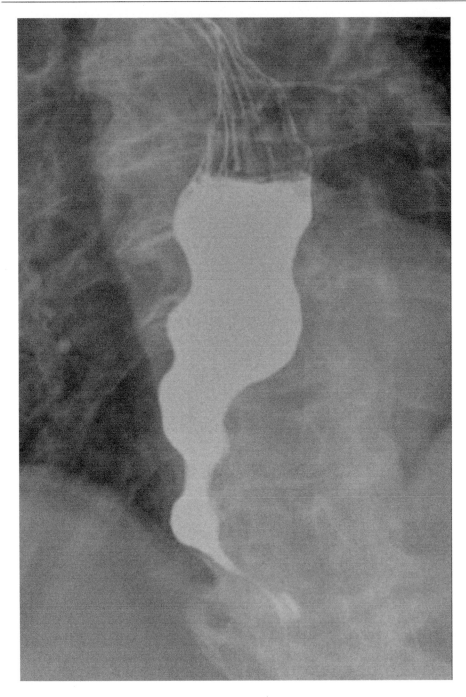

FIGURE 9.7

Clinical Information: 49-year-old man with long-standing clinical history of dysphagia, regurgitation and heartburn, empirically treated as 'gastritis and gastroesophageal reflux'.

Comment: The next three figures will show cases of very subtle, transient bird-beak signs that can be evident in just a few frames out of the 90–100 frames we acquire during morphodynamical examinations. While from a radiologic point of view these 'transient' signs are similar to the 'subtle' ones described before, because of the actual conformation and their being not easily detectable, they tend to be often found in early-stage disease, when even other suggestive findings are not clearly depicted. The case shown is Figure 9.7 is the easiest of the three 'transient' signs described in this chapter, because the presence of spasm clearly gives away that, at least, the oesophageal findings are not completely unremarkable. The evidence of low-degree dilation, along with spasm, points towards a spastic oesophageal motility disorder—the detection of the transient bird-beak sign confirms the presence of a type III achalasia.

Additional Findings: Dilation of low severity (3.6 cm) and spasm are noted. Stasis and hypotonia were not detected.

FBF Score and Staging: Bird-beak sign (+), Dilation (+), Hypotonia (–), Stasis (–), Spasm (+) = FBFs 4—type III Achalasia.

Tips: Transient bird-beak signs tend to be found in borderline, early-stage disease cases of all types of achalasia. The other findings related to oesophageal motility disorders might be either absent, as hypotonia and stasis in this case or present but subtle or confusing, as spasm in this case. The presence of a bird-beak sign in a spastic oesophagus, as in this case, changes the diagnosis from a blurry, non-specified spastic disease, to a type III achalasia. *Our tip in this kind of situation is to consider each motility disorder to be suspect for achalasia and to carefully look for the bird-beak sign*—of course, these are the cases in which high-resolution manometry is decisive. Our aim should be, however, to always send the patient to manometry with a suspect diagnosis as precise as possible.

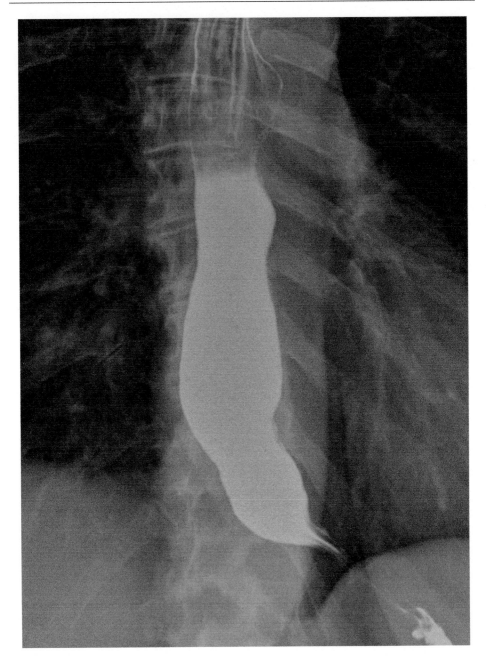

FIGURE 9.8

Clinical Information: 42-year-old woman with regurgitation and heartburn, occasional dysphagia. Patient specifies she has recently started to help herself to abundant mouthfuls of food during meals to relieve dysphagia.

Comment: The frame shown in Figure 9.8 demonstrates the beginning of the endoluminal stasis of the third bolus of barium at the distal oesophagus, above the LES, and the presence of a transient bird-beak sign—this is the only frame in this acquired sequence in which the sign is clearly visible, the GEJ tightly shut and not explorable in the others. The first two boluses had been, curiously enough, totally unremarkable. Dilation, hypotonia and stasis became apparent and were confirmed only at the five-minute timed barium film, configuring an early-stage type I achalasia. A static examination or, even worse, an examination not conducted properly, could have been easily passed as inconclusive.

Additional Findings: Dilation of low severity (3.3 cm), hypotonia and stasis were all noted, albeit quite late during the examination.

FBF Score and Staging: Bird-beak sign (+), Dilation (+), Hypotonia (+), Stasis (+), Spasm (−) = FBFs 8—type I Achalasia.

Tips: As stated before, 'transient' bird-beak signs are commonly found in early-stage disease of all three types. In this case, however, the bird beak was detected on just a couple of frames at the beginning of the third bolus, after a two completely unremarkable boluses—it can happen, in early-stage disease, that an examination might be completely or partially unremarkable or, at least, might be deemed as normal when findings are extremely subtle. Normal boluses might lower the level of attention of the examiner and prompt an early, guilty dismissal of the examination as negative. The detection of the bird beak and occasional GEJ tight closure at the live review during the examination forced us to give another, rather abundant bolus that remarkably failed to open the GEJ. The presence of findings suggestive for an early-stage type I achalasia became apparent at the five-minute timed barium film—the oesophagus spontaneously emptied on the seventh minute. Our suggestion, in these instances, is to carefully review the acquired frames live, one by one, to search for the bird-beak sign and be patient, wait at least five minutes, to obtain the appearance of other findings. Morphodynamic imaging is fundamental in these specific cases, because it allows subtle findings to eventually come out if we search for them.

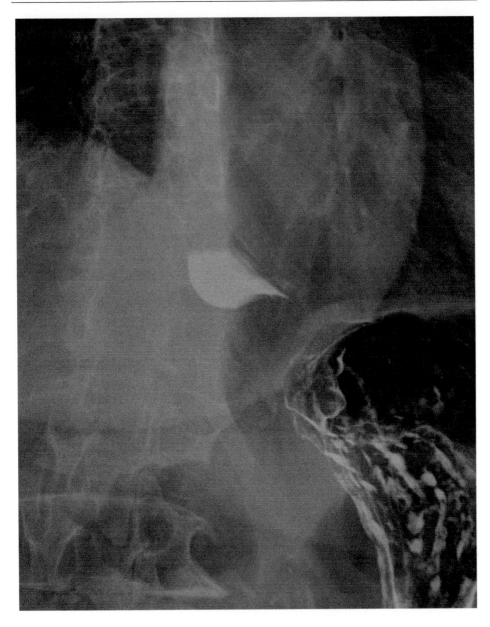

FIGURE 9.9

Clinical Information: 38-year-old man with odynophagia, regurgitation and heartburn.

Comment: The transient bird-beak sign in Figure 9.9 can clearly be seen on just three of the 102 frames making up the entire examination; those frames depict the exact moments some of the barium is allowed to pass into the gastric lumen.

Additional Findings: Dilation of low severity (3.2 cm), hypotonia and stasis were all noted, albeit quite late during the examination.

FBF Score and Staging: Bird-beak sign (+), Dilation (+), Hypotonia (+), Stasis (+), Spasm (–) = FBFs 8—type I Achalasia.

Tips: In this case, some signs of motility disease were evident from the beginning, especially the gradually worsening endoluminal stasis; others, including our bird-beak sign, were subtler: some mild degree of hypotonia became apparent along with the endoluminal stasis relatively soon, but dilation and the bird beak were found only after careful frame-by-frame observation and measuring. *Do give the appropriate amount of time and attention to every barium swallow you have the honour to report.*

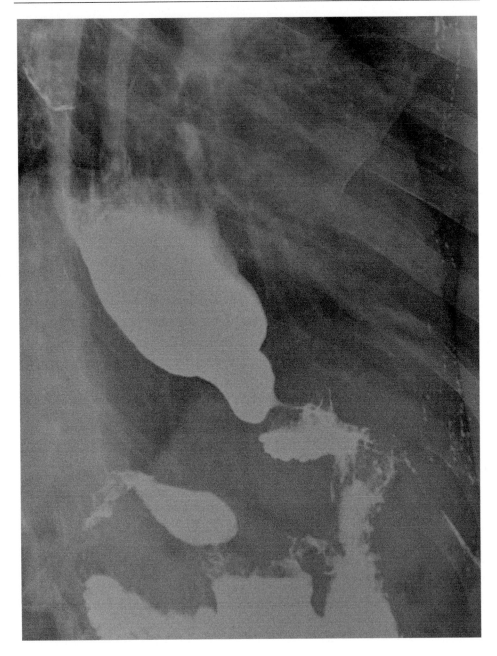

FIGURE 9.10

Clinical Information: 54-year-old woman with long-standing history of untreated dysphagia, odynophagia, regurgitation, coughing, heartburn and eating disorders, causing important weight loss, retreat from social life and psychological consequences.

Comment: This very peculiar type of bird-beak sign in Figure 9.10, with its thin, linear morphology, was noted, pretty much unchanged, in the vast majority of acquired frames. Quite resembling of the elongated/opening subtypes, it is almost exclusively found in severe atonic type I achalasia and is the radiologic translation of an extremely tight GEJ; we were not able to witness even a partial opening of the LES during our examination, which lasted more than 45 minutes. No food impaction was noted, because the patient had not been able to eat actual solid food for days; curiously enough, though, a discrete quantity of barium can be seen in the gastric, duodenal and jejunal lumen—small quantities of thin barium were able to pass through the LES after a few minutes, without forcing a valid opening.

Additional Findings: Severe dilation (6.7 cm), hypotonia and stasis were all noted.

FBF Score and Staging: Bird-beak sign (+), Dilation (+++), Hypotonia (+), Stasis (+), Spasm (−) = FBFs 12—type I Achalasia.

Tips: This subtype of the bird-beak or rat-tail sign should generally ring bells and point, along with other findings, towards a prompt diagnosis of severe atonic achalasia. *Sometimes, situations like these might need emergency treatment, so keep this in mind.* This specific patient was rapidly sent for an emergency PD and subsequently referred to get psychological help.

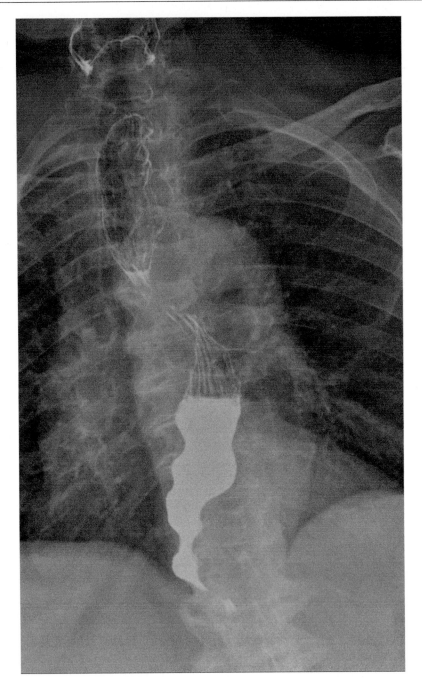

FIGURE 9.11

Clinical Information: 51-year-old man with dysphagia and chest pain.

Comment: Low-degree or grade I luminal dilations are present when the maximum climber of the lumen is between 3 and 4 cm. They are probably the easiest to miss, because slightly dilated lumina such as the one in Figure 9.11 (3.2 cm), might be passed as normal when not measured, especially in achalasia subtypes II and III.

Additional Findings: Bird-beak sign, stasis and spasm were all noted.

FBF Score and Staging: Bird-beak sign (+), Dilation (+), Hypotonia (−), Stasis (+), Spasm (+) = FBFs 6—type III Achalasia.

Tips: When suspecting oesophageal motility disorders, *always measure the maximum caliber of the oesophagus in each stack of images you acquire.* Do not hesitate to report even the slightest degree of dilation you might find.

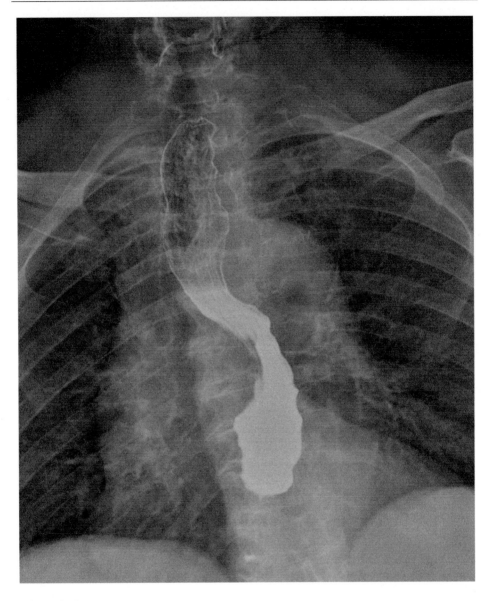

FIGURE 9.12

Clinical Information: 49-year-old man with dysphagia and weight loss.

Comment: A 3.8 cm, low-degree luminal dilation is shown in Figure 9.12. In a panpressurized lumen such as the one in this case, the actual luminal caliber might be very often underestimated, due to the peculiar condition found in type II achalasia. In fact, we found, in the whole examination, only a few frames clearly showing dilation.

Additional Findings: Bird-beak sign (not shown) and stasis were noted.

FBF Score and Staging: Bird-beak sign (+), Dilation (+), Hypotonia (−), Stasis (+), Spasm (−) = FBFs 6—type II Achalasia.

Tips: A good attitude towards detecting luminal dilation is measuring real-time during examinations, after each acquired sequence, especially in achalasia subtypes in which dilation might be subtler, such as subtypes II and III. This is of great help in forming a suspect diagnosis, also considering a bird-beak sign should be detected before dilation, and quickens the reporting process.

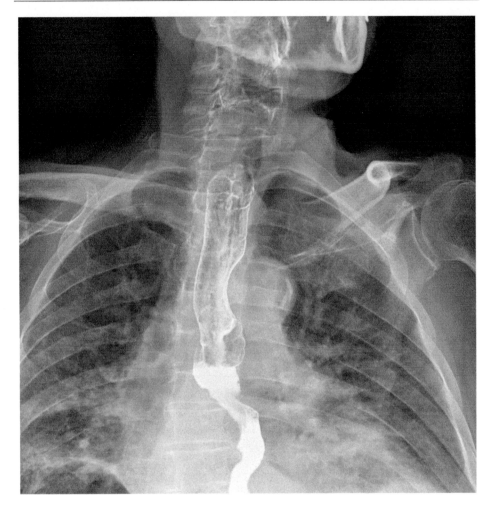

FIGURE 9.13

Clinical Information: 41-year-old woman with worsening dysphagia and eating disorders.

Comment: In this case, as often found in panpressurized and spastic achalasia, the lower two-thirds of the oesophagus are of normal caliber, albeit in presence of vigorous spasms; this generally tends to create an area of relatively lower pressure that end up being slightly dilated. A low-degree luminal dilation is found in Figure 9.13 (3.2 cm), at the paratracheal portion.

Additional Findings: Aortosclerosis and right parahilar disventilations.

FBF Score and Staging: Bird-beak sign (+), Dilation (+), Hypotonia (−), Stasis (+), Spasm (+) = FBFs 6—type III Achalasia.

Tips: Do not bypass luminal measuring in subtypes II and III and carefully examine each portion of the lumen, including the upper ones, which are more easily dilated in these cases.

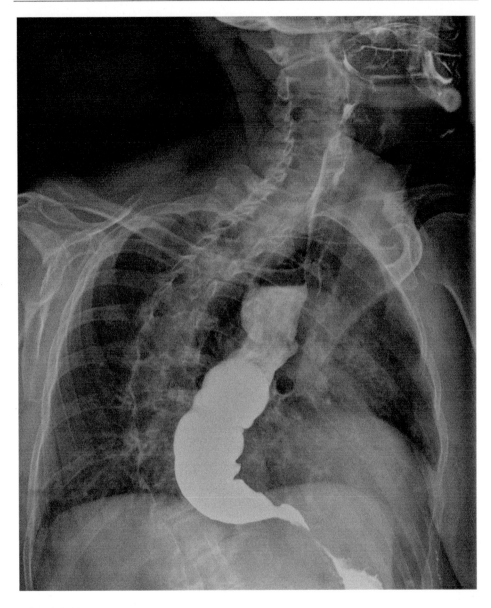

FIGURE 9.14

Clinical Information: 53-year-old man with history of untreated dysphagia, odynophagia and regurgitation.

Comment: A medium-degree dilation is present when the maximum luminal caliber measures between 4 and 6 cm. Figure 9.14 clearly demonstrates a medium-degree dilation (4.8 cm), affecting the lumen between the aortic and epiphrenal portions.

Additional Findings: Bird-beak sign, hypotonia, and stasis were all noted.

FBF Score and Staging: Bird-beak sign (+), Dilation (++), Hypotonia (+), Stasis (+), Spasm (−) = FBFs 10—type I Achalasia.

Tips: Medium-degree dilations tend to be easily detected. Measurements are generally best taken on AP or LL frames but can be obtained on oblique frames, when necessary, as in this case.

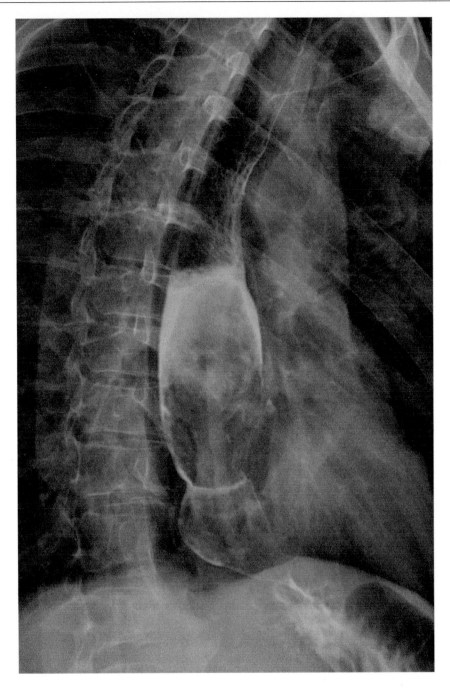

FIGURE 9.15

Clinical Information: 49-year-old woman with severe dysphagia/odynophagia and weight loss.

Comment: Diluted iodinated contrast was used in this case (Figure 9.15). Measurements might be trickier in these cases because the mucosal profile is generally thinner and retains less contrast than in classic barium swallows. A 4.7 cm luminal dilation is noted at the cardiac/epiphrenal portion.

Additional Findings: A Schatzki ring is noted at the epiphrenal portion of the oesophagus.

FBF Score and Staging: Bird-beak sign (+), Dilation (++), Hypotonia (+), Stasis (+), Spasm (−) = FBFs 10—type I Achalasia.

Tips: Sometimes dysphagia can be so dramatic that patients dread drinking barium in fear of bolus impaction. While the overall quality of examinations remains generally acceptable, a higher level of attention and number of frames per second are needed when using iodinated contrast.

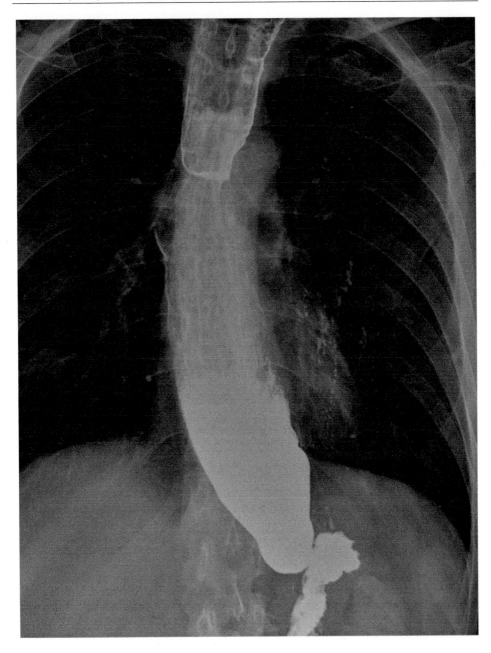

FIGURE 9.16

Clinical Information: 37-year-old man with mild but rapidly deteriorating dysphagia, regurgitation and heartburn.

Comment: A 5.4 cm luminal dilation is noted at the cardiac portion of the oesophagus (Figure 9.16).

Additional Findings: Bird-beak sign (not shown), hypotonia, and stasis were all noted.

FBF Score and Staging: Bird-beak sign (+), Dilation (++), Hypotonia (+), Stasis (+), Spasm (–) = FBFs 10—type I Achalasia.

Tips: Albeit luminal dilation is noted fairly easily and quickly when moderate or severe, its degree might sometimes change during the examination. When a mild dilation starts deteriorating into a moderate or severe one, measurements are best taken on the last acquired stacks, when luminal stasis has already kicked in. In this case, a moderate (>4 cm) dilation was noted in the last acquired sequence only.

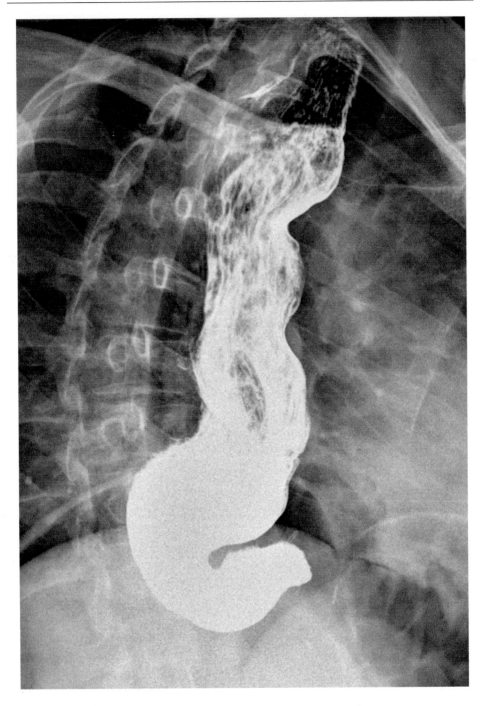

FIGURE 9.17

Clinical Information: 54-year-old woman with long-standing history of untreated dysphagia, odynophagia, regurgitation, coughing, heartburn and eating disorders, causing important weight loss, retreat from social life and psychological consequences.

Comment: Figure 9.17 clearly depicts an end-stage, atonic, and sigmoid oesophagus in type I achalasia. A 6.5 luminal dilation is noted at the paratracheal portion.

Additional Findings: Reactive changes to the mucosal profile are noted, along all classic hallmarks of atonic achalasia.

FBF Score and Staging: Bird-beak sign (+), Dilation (+++), Hypotonia (+), Stasis (+), Spasm (–) = FBFs 12—type I Achalasia.

Tips: A sigmoid oesophagus is inevitably synonymous with end-stage, FBFs 12, type I disease. Albeit easily diagnosed, careful detection of signs and measurements is needed—these patients often undergo post-therapeutic/post-surgical follow-ups and eventual improvements in oesophageal outflow could be evident only by comparing measurements.

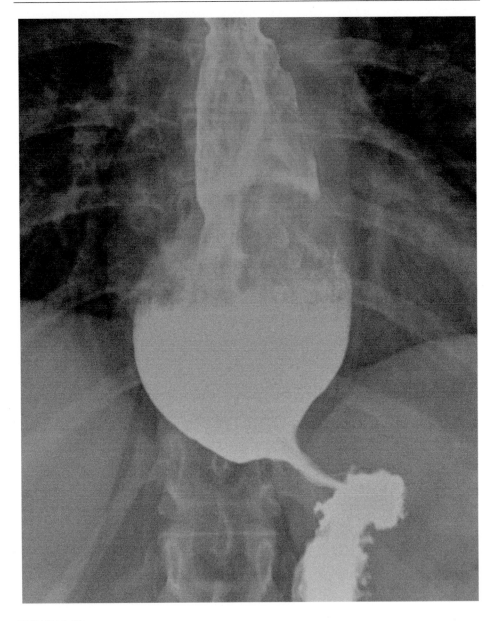

FIGURE 9.18

Comment: A 6.8 cm luminal dilation is noted at the cardiac portion, in a severely hypotonic oesophagus (Figure 9.18).

Additional Findings: Reactive changes to the mucosal profile were noted.

FBF Score and Staging: Bird-beak sign (+), Dilation (+++), Hypotonia (+), Stasis (+), Spasm (−) = FBFs 12—type I Achalasia.

Tips: The measurement to take account of when reporting should be the longest detectable in the acquired frames. Always choose and state the exact portion of dilated lumen; this information is crucial, as already said, for monitoring patients after therapy.

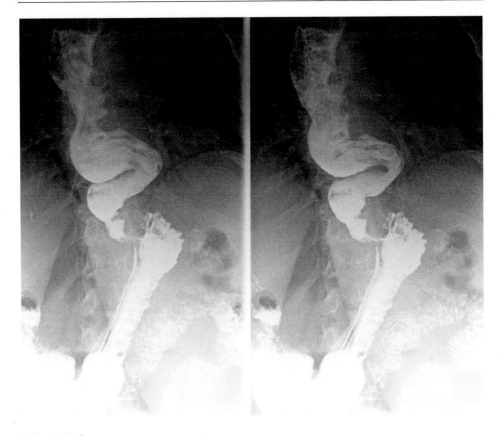

FIGURE 9.19

Clinical Information: 49-year-old man with severe dysphagia, regurgitation, and heartburn, almost completely retired from social life. Previous gastric surgery unrelated to achalasia.

Comment: A sigmoid, end-stage atonic type I oesophagus is shown in Figure 9.19. A severely dilated lumen is noted in various portions, the largest caliber being 6.9 at the aortobronchial portion.

Additional Findings: Reactive changes to the mucosal profile, bird-beak sign, hypotonia, and stasis were all noted.

FBF Score and Staging: Bird-beak sign (+), Dilation (+++), Hypotonia (+), Stasis (+), Spasm (−) = FBFs 12—type I Achalasia.

Tips: Do not underestimate the dilation of the proximal portions of the oesophagus and duly measure each time the caliber is abnormal.

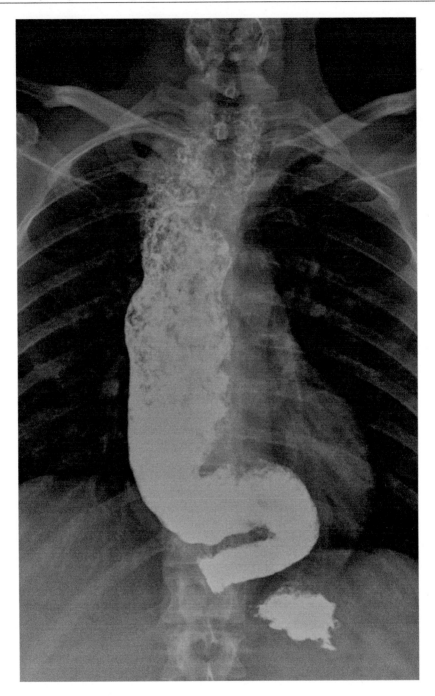

FIGURE 9.20

Clinical Information: 51-year-old woman with known but untreated severe achalasia and classic symptoms.

Comment: Severe sigmoid atonic achalasia, with a tightly closed LES and severe dilation (6.1 cm), is shown in Figure 9.20.

Additional Findings: Reactive changes to the mucosal profile due to irritation.

FBF Score and Staging: Bird-beak sign (+, evident only very late into the examination), Dilation (+++), Hypotonia (+), Stasis (+), Spasm (–) = FBFs 12—type I Achalasia.

Tips: The sight of a sigmoid oesophagus might suggest an automatic diagnosis of severe dilation (>6 cm)—this is not always true and albeit the clinical difference between calibers around the 6 cm hallmark is almost none; correct measurements are usually needed for follow-ups. In this specific case, a diagnosis of severe dilation was very narrow.

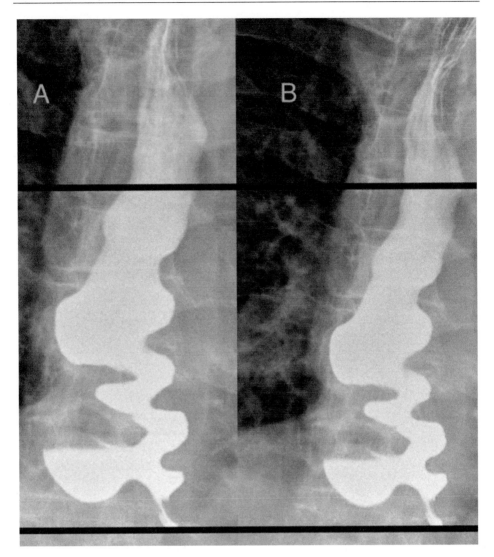

FIGURE 9.21

Comment: Figures 9.21A and B were taken five minutes apart, the latter being the static timed barium control. The barium columns do not look significantly different, with the height in Figure 9.21B being non-significantly lower than the other; the comparable constant higher levels suggest the presence of stasis.

Additional Findings: Bird-beak sign, mild dilation, and spasm were all noted.

FBF Score and Staging: Bird-beak sign (+), Dilation (+), Hypotonia (−), Stasis (+), Spasm (+) = FBFs 4—type III Achalasia.

Tips: As stated in previous chapters, barium column heights are measured considering the LES and the upper level on the frame taken at time 0 as a standard. A difference of barium height of less than 10% of the total is considered non-significant and heights might be considered as comparable, as in this case.

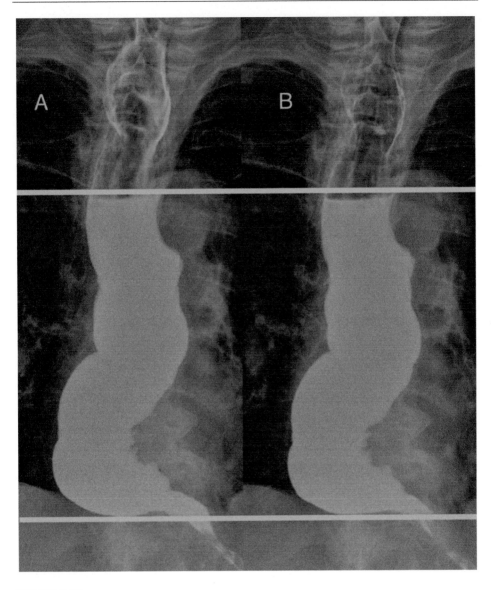

FIGURE 9.22

Comment: Figures 9.22A and B were taken five minutes apart, the latter being the static timed barium control. The barium columns look almost identical, with comparable constant higher levels, suggesting the presence of stasis.

Additional Findings: Bird-beak sign, moderate dilation and hypotonia were all noted.

FBF Score and Staging: Bird-beak sign (+), Dilation (++), Hypotonia (+), Stasis (+), Spasm (−) = FBFs 10—type I Achalasia.

Tips: When at five minutes we have not only comparable column heights, but almost completely identical frames, it could be worth acquiring a ten-minute control frame as well to assess severity and for follow-up information.

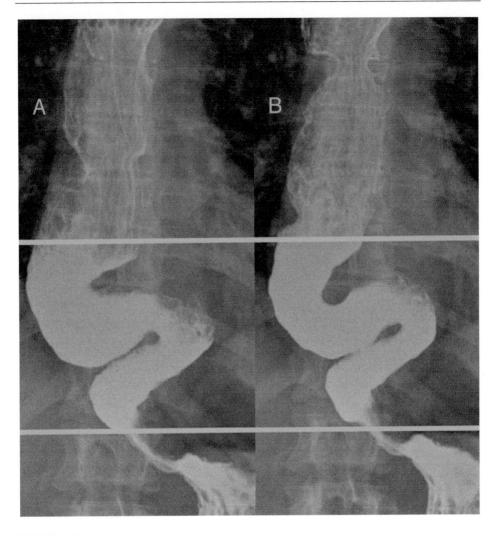

FIGURE 9.23

Comment: Figures 9.23A and B were taken ten minutes apart, the latter being the static timed barium control. The barium columns look almost identical in this case as well.

Additional Findings: Bird-beak sign, severe dilation and hypotonia were all noted.

FBF Score and Staging: Bird-beak sign (+), Dilation (+++), Hypotonia (+), Stasis (+), Spasm (−) = FBFs 12—type I Achalasia.

Tips: In the case of sigmoid achalasia, we suggest taking the control film at ten or even 15 minutes, considering the relative severity of these end-stage diseases.

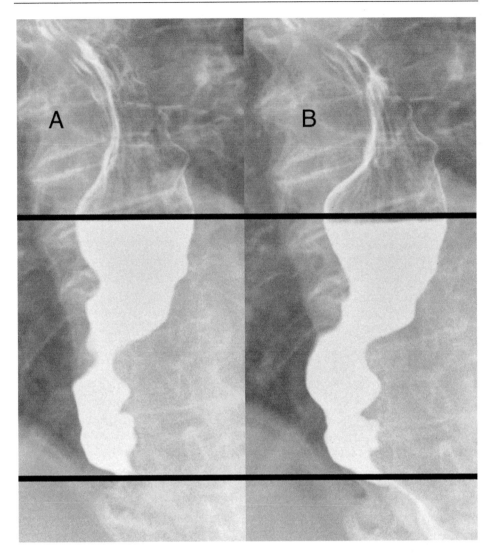

FIGURE 9.24

Comment: Figures 9.24A and B were taken five minutes apart, the latter being the static timed barium control. The barium columns look almost identical in this panpressurized lumen.

Additional Findings: Bird-beak sign and moderate dilation were noted.

FBF Score and Staging: Bird-beak sign (+), Dilation (++), Hypotonia (−), Stasis (+), Spasm (−) = FBFs 8—type II Achalasia.

Tips: Sometimes, especially in subtypes II-III disease, one might be tempted to skip the five-minute control when stasis is evident at fluoroscopy after a minute or two. Duly acquire the five-minute control film always, as sometimes it is the only frame we need to compare in follow-up.

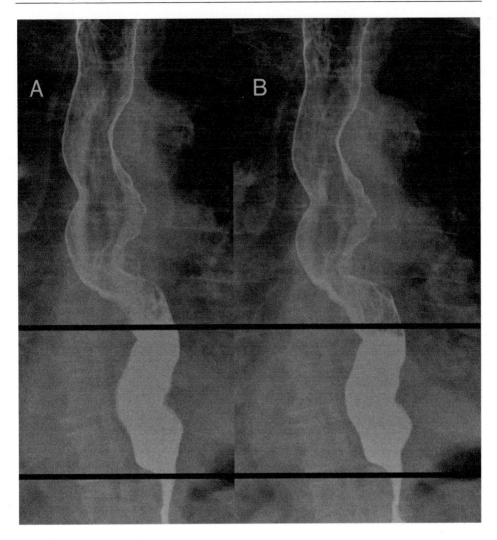

FIGURE 9.25

Comment: Figures 9.25A and B were taken eight minutes apart, the latter being the static timed barium control. The barium columns look almost identical, in a rather spastic lumen.

Additional Findings: Bird-beak sign, moderate dilation and spasm were all noted.

FBF Score and Staging: Bird-beak sign (+), Dilation (++), Hypotonia (–), Stasis (+), Spasm (+) = FBFs 6—type III Achalasia.

Tips: Barium columns do not need to be high to detect stasis. Once we start acquiring frames and oesophageal outflow insufficiency becomes clear, sometimes this happening straight away after the start, we have to choose which frame we want to use as a standard. Figure 9.25A was chosen during a partial opening and sudden re-closure of the LES, which basically remained unchanged for several minutes afterwards. This search for the right frame and its time of execution might sometimes not be easy or quick—it might happen that the control film is taken at six, eight, as in this case, or ten minutes; it is crucial to state the right timing, because on a follow-up examination, this patient must always have his control film taken at the exact timing, eight minutes.

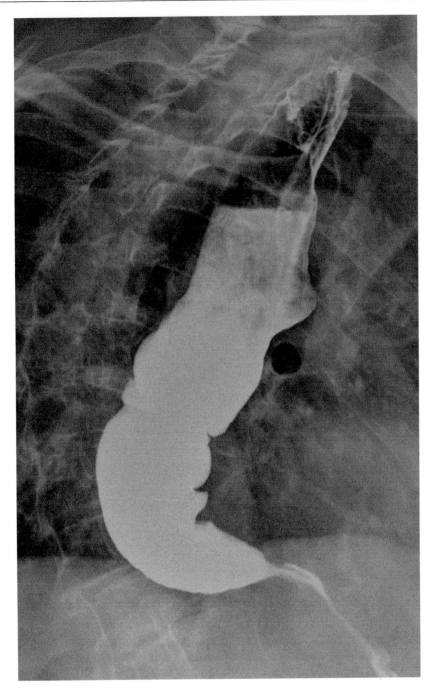

FIGURE 9.26

Comment: Hypotonia is noted in Figure 9.26, in the form of multiple folds evident at the lower half of the oesophageal body, signalling the presence of areas of reduced or absent peristalsis which can, if left untreated, evolve into an end-stage disease.

Additional Findings: Bird-beak sign, severe dilation, and stasis were all noted.

FBF Score and Staging: Bird-beak sign (+), Dilation (+++), Hypotonia (+), Stasis (+), Spasm (−) = FBFs 12—type I Achalasia.

Tips: The different degrees of hypotonia and peristaltic incoordination might be difficult to assess on static frames. That is why we suggest you concentrate on acquiring a dedicated stack including most of the oesophagus, as in Figure 9.26, using a high number of frames per second, generally in the oblique projection. Peristaltic failure, folds and non-propulsive contractions will be more evident when carefully reviewed.

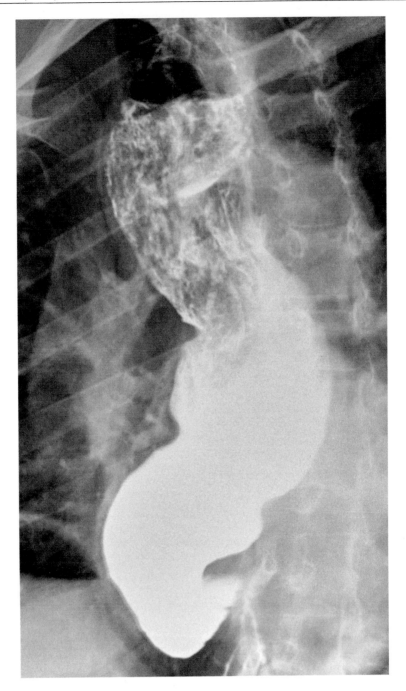

FIGURE 9.27

Comment: Figure 9.27 shows a severely hypotonic oesophageal lumen, with initial folding, suggestive of a near end-stage evolution and mostly non-propulsive peristalsis.

Additional Findings: Bird-beak sign, severe dilation, hypotonia and stasis were all noted.

FBF Score and Staging: Bird-beak sign (not shown, +), Dilation (+++), Hypotonia (+), Stasis (+), Spasm (−) = FBFs 12—type I Achalasia.

Tips: A marker of the severity of the peristaltic impairment is the concurrent stasis. We chose this frame specifically because it depicts the stratification of the luminal content, with barium mostly present at the lower portions of the oesophagus and more diluted content evident upstream—this generally happens in severely hypotonic or atonic diseases.

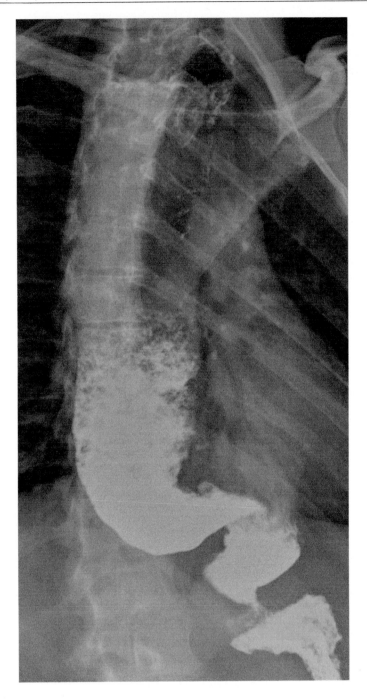

FIGURE 9.28

Comment: A severely atonic, sigmoid type I disease oesophagus is shown in Figure 9.28. Only occasional, often non-peristaltic contractions were observed.

Additional Findings: Bird-beak sign, severe dilation, hypotonia and stasis were all noted.

FBF Score and Staging: Bird-beak sign (+), Dilation (+++), Hypotonia (+), Stasis (+), Spasm (−) = FBFs 12—type I Achalasia.

Tips: This form of disease is a highly severe one, because peristalsis is limited to a bare, often non-propulsive minimum. Occasional LES opening shows some emptying of barium in the stomach taking place, some 27 minutes after the start of the examination. In these patients, it might be worth waiting enough time, monitoring with fluoroscopy and acquiring a static frame when the actual emptying happens—this is done always for follow-up purposes, and time of emptying should be clearly stated.

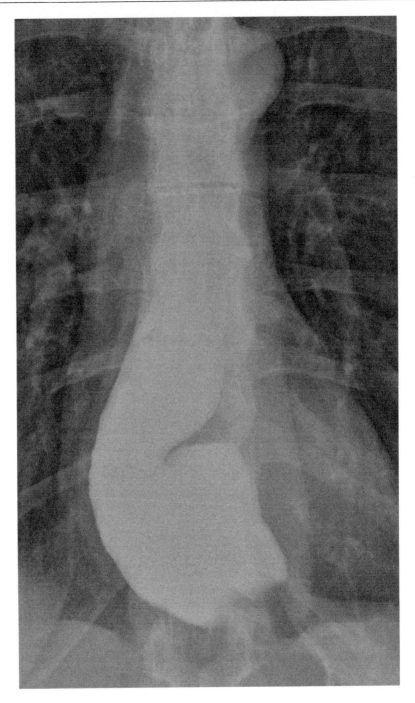

FIGURE 9.29

Comment: Figure 9.29 shows a moderately hypotonic oesophageal lumen, with an epiphrenic outpouching, with little evidence of propulsive peristalsis.

Additional Findings: Bird-beak sign (not shown), moderate dilation, hypotonia and stasis were all noted. An epiphrenic diverticulum is evident.

FBF Score and Staging: Bird-beak sign (not shown, +), Dilation (++), Hypotonia (+), Stasis (+), Spasm (–) = FBFs 10—type I Achalasia.

Tips: Epiphrenic diverticula are generally false pulsion outpouchings located at the lower end of the esophagus, almost inevitably but motility disorders such as achalasia. This happens when the increasingly high endoluminal pressure cannot be overcome by the oesophageal body, which can either evolve towards a spastic, or a hypotonic state, such as in this case.

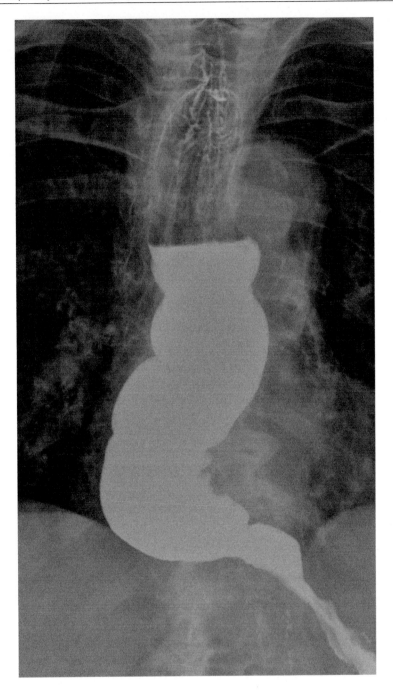

FIGURE 9.30

Comment: Figure 9.30 shows a mildly hypotonic oesophageal body, with folding noted at the lower half.

Additional Findings: Bird-beak sign, moderate dilation and stasis were all noted.

FBF Score and Staging: Bird-beak sign (+), Dilation (++), Hypotonia (+), Stasis (+), Spasm (–) = FBFs 10—type I Achalasia.

Tips: The evidence of folding, especially when the motility impairment is mild or moderate, should be pointed out in the additional notes, as it is considered a marker for unfavourable course of disease.

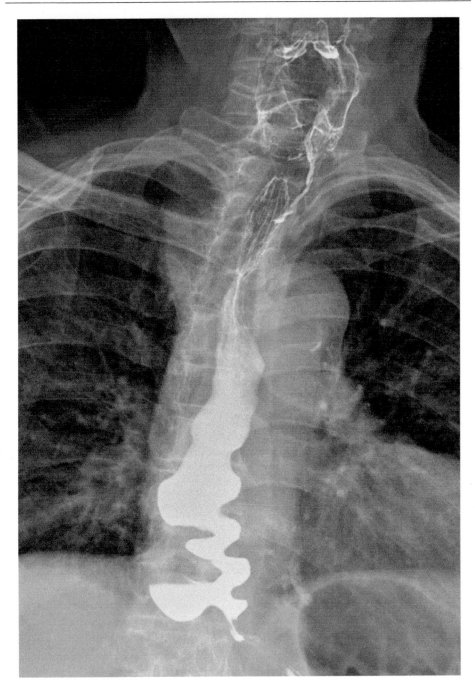

FIGURE 9.31

Comment: Figure 9.31 shows a blatant case of spastic, subtype III achalasia. Until not very long ago, probably until HR manometry was introduced into clinical practice, situations like this one might have easily been dismissed as a 'corkscrew oesophagus' or, vaguely, as a 'spastic motility disorder', mainly because the picture clinicians and, sadly enough, many radiologists have in mind when thinking about achalasia is generally that of atonic achalasia. The corkscrew pattern is of course the main feature of a spastic oesophagus but, at the same time, other signs suggestive for achalasia are present.

Additional Findings: An epiphrenic diverticulum is noted, arising from the right aspect of the oesophageal wall.

FBF Score and Staging: Bird-beak sign (+), Dilation (++), Hypotonia (−), Stasis (+), Spasm (+) = FBFs 6—type III Achalasia.

Tips: The presence of spasms is easily highlighted here by the presence of both narrowed and dilated luminal portions. The difference between a nonspecific spastic disorder and a spastic achalasia is the presence of a hypertonic LES (bird-beak sign), dilated portions, end-liminal stasis of contrast and, of course, spasms—look for these signs when in presence of a spastic oesophagus.

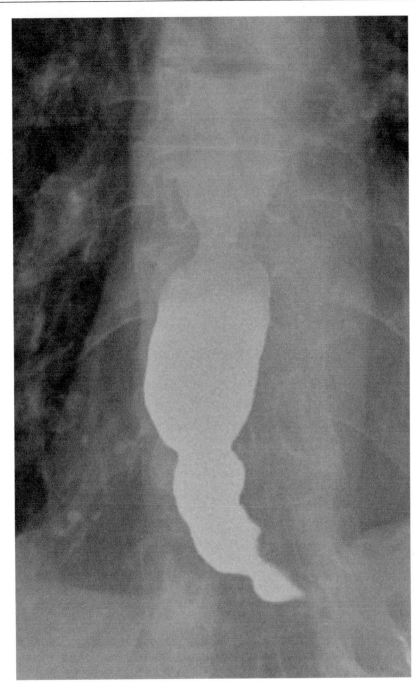

FIGURE 9.32

Comment: Figure 9.32 shows the presence of constant, consecutive alternated portions of dilated and narrowed lumen, compatible with spasm.

Additional Findings: Severe dilation (6.7 cm), hypotonia and stasis were all noted.

FBF Score and Staging: Bird-beak sign (+), Dilation (+), Hypotonia (−), Stasis (+), Spasm (+) = FBFs 4—type III Achalasia.

Tips: Do not expect spasm to always be extreme in its depiction. End-stage, tortuous cases are generally the evolution of milder situations, such as the one pictured here. Spasm can be reported every time the luminal caliber is altered by the presence of narrowed and dilated luminal portions, which tend to spastically remain fixed in this position.

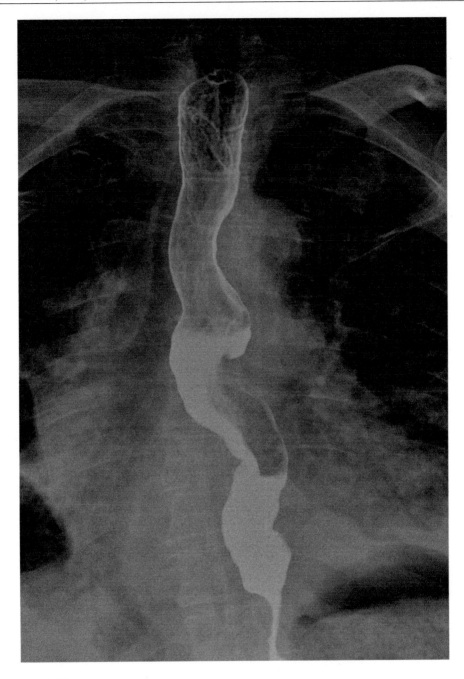

FIGURE 9.33

Comment: Figure 9.33 shows the presence of a spastically tortuous oesophagus, revolving around its own axis, with focal stasis at the aortobronchial portion, where a saccular outpouching is noted, on the left aspect of the mucosal profile. This fixed, wide-radius corkscrew appearance is another typical feature considered a spasm.

Additional Findings: Bird-beak sign, mild dilation and stasis were noted.

FBF Score and Staging: Bird-beak sign (+), Dilation (+), Hypotonia (−), Stasis (+), Spasm (+) = FBFs 4—type III Achalasia.

Tips: Regardless of morphology, an oesophageal body fixed in its appearance should always be considered spastic.

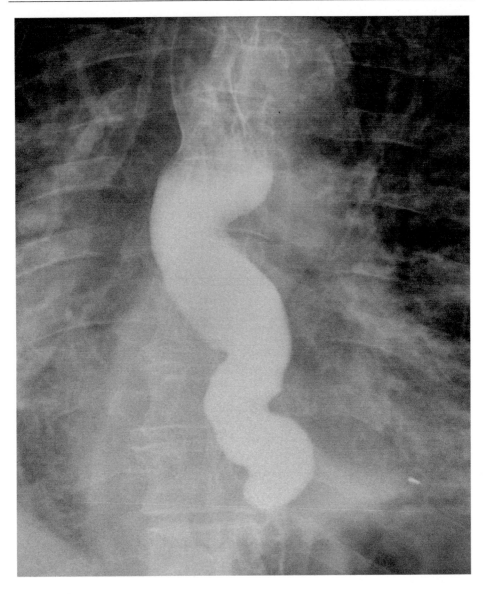

FIGURE 9.34

Comment: Figure 9.34 shows another wide-range corkscrew spastic appearance, at a late stage during the examination. In this frame, a tightly closed LES is evident, with severe upstream stasis and moderate dilation, in a rather fixed oesophageal body.

Additional Findings: A surgical clip can be found at the gastric fundus.

FBF Score and Staging: Bird-beak sign (+), Dilation (++), Hypotonia (−), Stasis (+), Spasm (+) = FBFs 6—type III Achalasia.

Tips: Albeit a spastic oesophagus's appearance might change a little in time, especially due to worsening stasis—this helping in measuring a more realistic caliber—the overall revolving around the axis should remain unchanged, when spasm is present.

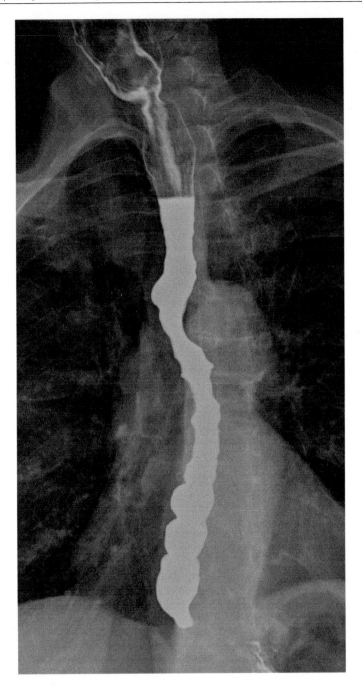

FIGURE 9.35

Comment: Multiple focal spastic, fixed contractions can be seen in this frame, along with severe stasis, upstream of a tightly clenched LES (Figure 9.35).

Additional Findings: Bird-beak sign, mild dilation and stasis were all noted.

FBF Score and Staging: Bird-beak sign (+), Dilation (+), Hypotonia (−), Stasis (+), Spasm (+) = FBFs 4—type III Achalasia.

Tips: This 'rosary bead' appearance is very often in common with spastic, non-achalasic motility disorders and is often dismissed as pathologic but unspecific. However, even though the presence of achalasia can be eventually confirmed at HR manometry, its presence has to be suspected in any case of motility disorder showing oesophageal outflow impairments and LES disfunction, as in this case. In these cases, reporting forms as ours can be of great help.

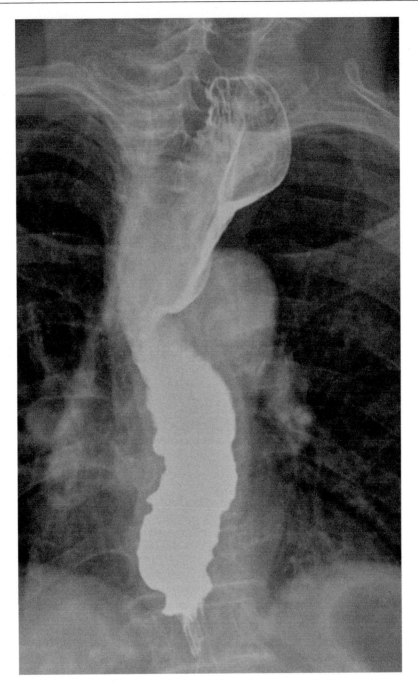

FIGURE 9.36

Comment: Figure 9.36 clearly depicts the hallmarks of a subtype II, panpressurized oesophagus, with subtle, frequent mostly unpropulsive peristaltic contractions typically affecting the lower two-thirds of the oesophageal body. Even though our approach to subtype II is a diagnosis by exclusion of subtypes I and III, it is important that each subtype should be recognized straight away, even when subtle.

Additional Findings: Bird-beak sign, moderate dilation and stasis are all noted.

FBF Score and Staging: Bird-beak sign (+), Dilation (++), Hypotonia (−), Stasis (+), Spasm (−) = FBFs 8—type II Achalasia.

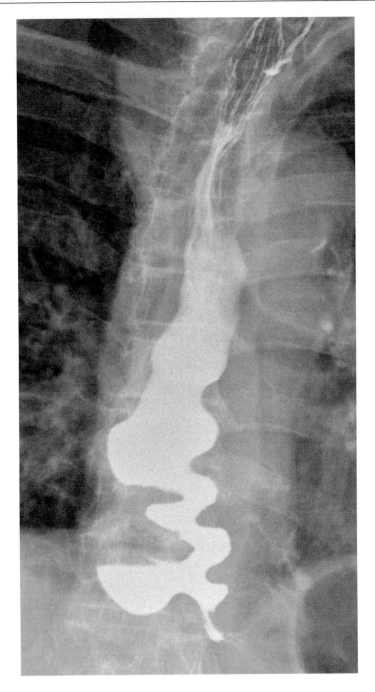

FIGURE 9.37

Comment: Epiphrenic diverticula are, in general, a rather uncommon sight, with a prevalence ranging between 0.015% and 2% worldwide (Figure 9.37). They are more easily detected in males between the sixth and seventh decades of life. They are false, pulsion diverticula arising from the last 10 cm of the oesophagus, above the diaphragm and are usually caused by alterations in endoluminal pressure, such as those present in all three subtypes of achalasia and other oesophageal motility disorders. It is easier, then, even though still very rare, to find such diverticula in patients with achalasia. When in presence of such findings, it is crucial not to take measurements regarding lumen dilation at the level of the diverticulum as, technically, the diverticulum is not part of the lumen.

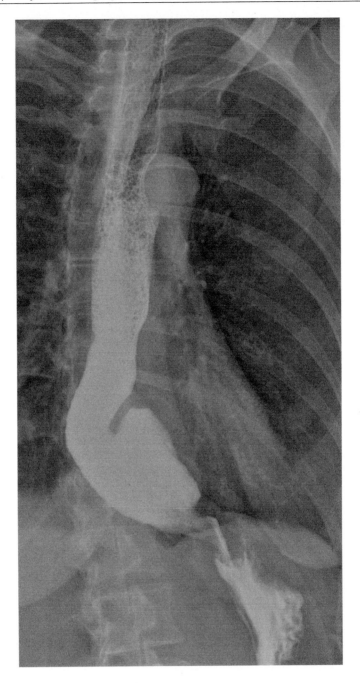

FIGURE 9.38

Comment: Another classic epiphrenic diverticulum found in a low-grade type I achalasia, along with other typical findings such as the bird-beak sign, stasis and lumen dilation (Figure 9.38). Mucosal profile irregularity, suggestive for reactive esophagitis, is noted at the aortic and proximal portions of the oesophagus.

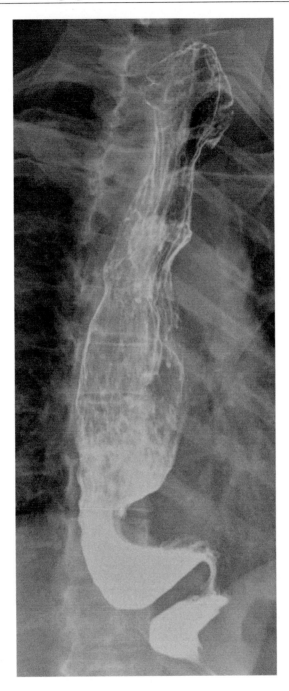

FIGURE 9.39

Comment: Mucosal profile irregularity and reactive changes are extremely common in achalasia and tend to be more severe in patients with moderate to end-stage disease, generally depending on, and directly proportional to the endoluminal stasis of bolus (Figure 9.39). The presence of such findings has to be reported in the notes on the report, as these findings are generally correlated to pain or other uncomfortable symptoms that need specific treatment.

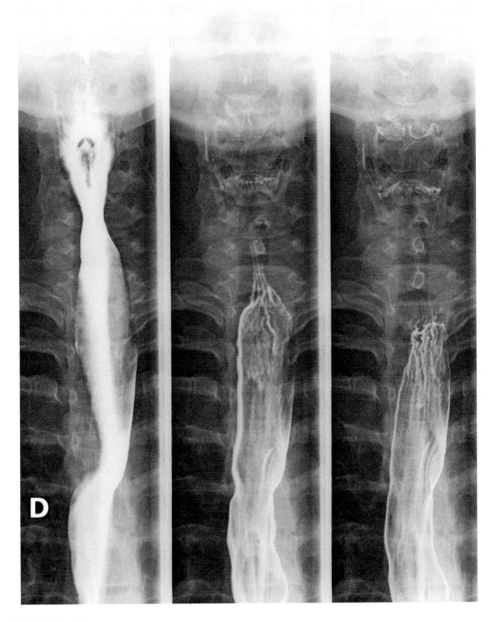

FIGURE 9.40

Comment: Reactive changes due to bolus endoluminal stasis generally determine a thickening and promote irregularity of the oesophageal mucosal profile (Figure 9.40). A plicar pattern vaguely resembling that of the gastric lumen is noted, both at the level of the stasis and oesophageal portions above. These signs are commonly associated with chest pain, regurgitation and heartburn.

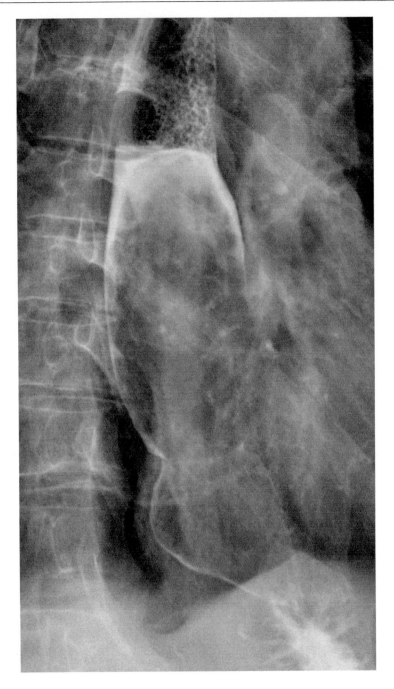

FIGURE 9.41

Comment: It is worth going back to the Schatzki ring noted a few pages back. It is generally thought of something totally unrelated to achalasia, but it is not uncommon that patients initially referred for suspected achalasia actually end up having a Schatzki ring. A relatively unknown entity, a Schatzki ring is a narrow, thin layer of mucosa, painted with contrast at barium swallow, generally found in the lower half of the oesophagus and seen as a response to reflux and endoluminal inflammation, which can cause even severe dysphagia. A correct identification of such entity is mandatory—the patient of the case pictured on Figure 9.41 had been misinterpreted for quite some time, and never treated, before arriving to our practice.

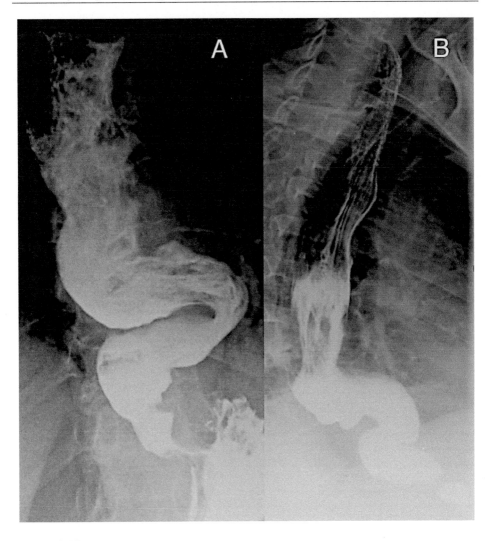

FIGURE 9.42

Comment: Figure 9.42 shows the same patient, with a sigmoid end-stage atonic subtype I achalasia, before (A) and after (B) two repetitions of PD, some 12 weeks after the beginning of the treatment. While, in this case, there is no substantial difference at the GEJ—considering generally patients show a mean caliber improvement of 6 mm at this level—a net decrease in luminal caliber and an overall better oesophageal outflow—confirmed by the patient himself—are noted. Even though the subtype I diagnosis will not and cannot change, the previous basal FBFs of 12, dropped to 10, due to changes in luminal caliber—another sign of improvement and therapy efficacy.

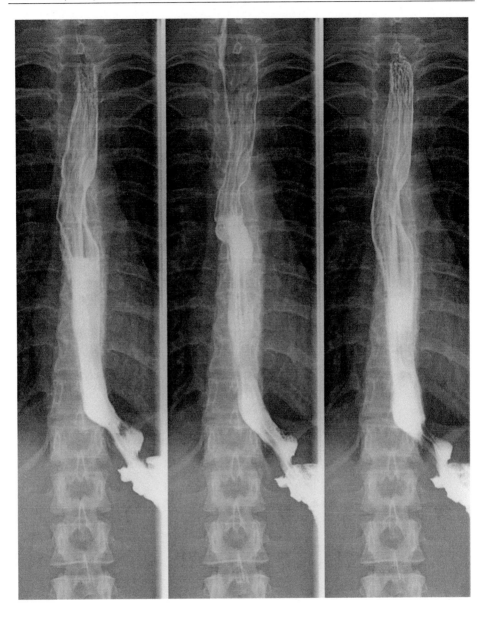

FIGURE 9.43

Comment: Figure 9.43 shows a common combination of treatments, Peroral Endoscopic Myotomy and Fundoplication. POEM, as seen before, is a rapidly emerging and equally effective alternative to Heller myotomy, which aims at the creation of a submucosal tunnel to reach and alter the integrity of the inner circular muscular bundle at the LES, while preserving the integrity of the outer longitudinal muscular layer, to lower endoluminal pressure at this level; sometimes this results in the creation of a gastroesophageal reflux condition of varying severity—that is why, as in this case, POEM usually coupled with protective fundoplication is the POEM+F combination. No bird-beak sign nor stasis are noted in Figure 9.43 as a result of POEM+F; mild dilation and esophagitis can be seen in the upper two-thirds of the lumen.

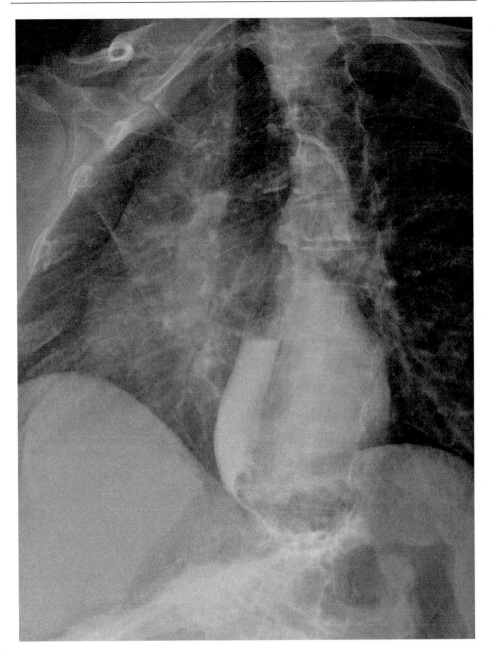

FIGURE 9.44

Clinical Information and Comment: The patient examined in Figure 9.44 is a 54-year-old male who experienced a gradually worsening dysphagia during the last six months, with odynophagia, chest pain that resulted in a weight loss of almost 10 kgs. Initially seen in our clinical GI practice, he was referred to us with a working diagnosis of achalasia, albeit the possible presence of malignancy was not excluded, of course: EGD had already been planned before barium swallow. It was clear from the beginning of the examination that we were not observing a case of achalasia: albeit something resembling a bird-beak sign can be seen, the tapering of the lumen is not gradual and the mucosal profile is markedly irregular, especially on the left aspect—a nodular oesophageal mass was, in fact, detected at EGD, with biopsies taken at the same time; a histologic diagnosis of oesophageal squamous carcinoma was confirmed later in the same week. Notably, however, all the signs related to achalasia were absent: the lumen caliber was normal, with no barium stasis noted. No alterations of the regular peristalsis, such as hypotonia or spasms, were observed.

9.45 FURTHER READING

Csendes A, Braghetto I, Henriquez A, Cortes C. Late results of prospective randomized study comparing forceful dilatation and oesophagomyotomy in patients with achalasia. *Gut.* 1989;30:299–304.

Ekberg O, Feinberg MJ. Altered swallowing function in elderly patients without dysphagia: radiologic findings in 56 cases. *Am J Roentgenol.* 1991;156:1181–4.

Liang CY, Lin MS. Images in clinical medicine: achalasia. *N Engl J Med* 2009;360:801.

Milas M, Hunter JG. Image of the month: achalasia. *Arch Surg* 2001;136:963–4.

Ott DJ, Richter JE, Chen YM, Wu WC, Gelfand DW, Castell DO. Esophageal radiography and manometry: correlation in 172 patients with dysphagia. *Am J Roentgenol.* 1987;149:307–11.

Schima W, Ryan JM, Harisinghani M, et al. Radiographic detection of achalasia: diagnostic accuracy of videofluoroscopy. *Clin Radiol.* 1998;53:372–5.

Conclusions

10

Giovanni Fontanella

Contents

10.1 FINAL CONSIDERATIONS

These last few lines mark the end of this volume dedicated to achalasia, a quite rare but, at times, profoundly devastating disease, with a huge impact on the daily routine, psychological wellness and overall quality of life. Although, as already hinted at the beginning of this chapter, the disease is actually infrequent, with an incidence standing at a pretty low 0.5–1.2 per 100,000, its striking radiologic features are to be instantly recognised even at a basic diagnostic level by a generic, non-subspecialised observer, and the aim of this book is to shed light on a topic that is often confined to a couple of lines in radiology books. The attention to fine details and the careful reporting and staging of the disease we described in this volume are the hallmarks of our way of interpreting our role as radiologists in the wider universe of medicine; of course, this pedantic approach to achalasia and, of course, all pharyngo-œsophageal disorders diagnosable with barium swallow, is welcomed even in non-specialised centers, but has been designed for, and finds its complete realisation in specialised centres, in which the patients are taken care of from the clinical examination, radiologic and instrumental evaluations, until the right therapeutic pathway is chosen. Centres devoted to swallowing and upper GI diseases are not, however, equally distributed and accessible to patients everywhere, and this makes diagnosing achalasia even more difficult, as in non-specialised institutions established care paths for such patients might not be in place or, even worse, there might not be enough expertise to correctly diagnose or treat the disease. That is why the existence of multidisciplinary teams and approach are mandatory: patients may end up not correctly diagnosed and staged, then 'contended' between gastroenterologists and surgeons—I can unfortunately recall at least a couple of such unfortunate cases. This is inconvenient and should not happen. Specialists involved in such kind of disease—gastroenterologists, surgeons, radiologists, paramedics—have to understand, accept their role in the care path not overdoing it, communicating with each

DOI: 10.1201/9781003320302-10

other in a clear and standardised way; that is why we insist on planning MDT meetings and on the importance of structured, standardised reporting. Our humble effort with this volume is not, in fact, intended just to enhance the role of radiology in the diagnostic process of achalasia; we are fully aware and grateful that the technological improvements have been more on the side of manometry and that high-resolution manometry is, up until today, the gold standard for the diagnosis and staging of achalasia. However, at the same time, our radiological research aimed at revamping a technique that is often misused or considered obsolete. Morphodynamic imaging has demonstrated to be of crucial support in dubious cases and a valid alternative to manometry when this is not readily available. Moreover, notwithstanding the huge role of high-resolution manometry in the post-therapeutic and evolutive follow-ups, morphodynamical analysis might be of incredible help in this setting as well, because it simply gives back morphologic data that are totally absent in manometry; in our experience, the visual approach to achalasia with barium swallow, before and after therapy, is generally preferred by surgeons.

Our hope is that, not only our experience with achalasia, but our whole integrated vision of medicine, too, can be transmitted through these pages to the readers.

Avellino, 17 March 2022
Giovanni Fontanella, MD FRSA

10.2 FURTHER READING

Andolfi, C., Baffy, G., & Fisichella, P. M. (2018). Whose patient is it? The path to multidisciplinary management of achalasia. *Journal of Surgical Research*, *228*, 8–13. https://doi.org/10.1016/j.jss.2018.02.047

Fontanella, G. (2021). A proposal for a new prognostic grading system in achalasia using dynamic barium swallow: The FBF score. *EMJ Radiology*, *2*(1), 34–6. Abstract Review.

O'Neill, O. M., Johnston, B. T., & Coleman, H. G. (2013). Achalasia: a review of clinical diagnosis, epidemiology, treatment and outcomes. *World Journal of Gastroenterology*, *19*(35), 5806–12. https://doi.org/10.3748/wjg.v19.i35.5806

Index

Note: Numbers in *italics* indicate figures and numbers in **bold** indicate tables on the corresponding page.